Clinical Handbook for Kozier & Erb's Fundamentals of Nursing

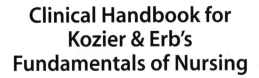

Clinical Handbook for Kozier & Erb's Fundamentals of Nursing

Concepts, Process, and Practice

EIGHTH EDITION

Berman • Snyder

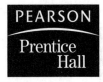

PEARSON

Prentice Hall

Upper Saddle River, New Jersey 07458

Library of Congress Cataloging-in-Publication data on file with the Library of Congress.

Pearson Prentice Hall™ is a trademark of Pearson Education, Inc.
Pearson® is a registered trademark of Pearson plc
Prentice Hall® is a registered trademark of Pearson Education, Inc.

Pearson Education Ltd.
Pearson Education Singapore Pte. Ltd.
Pearson Education Canada, Ltd.
Pearson Education—Japan
Pearson Education Australia Pty. Limited
Pearson Education North Asia Ltd.
Pearson Educación de Mexico, S. A. de C.V.
Pearson Education Malaysia Pte. Ltd.
Pearson Education, Inc., Upper Saddle River, New Jersey

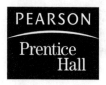

10 9 8 7 6 5 4 3 2 1
ISBN-10: 0-13-188933-8
ISBN-13: 978-0-13-188933-0

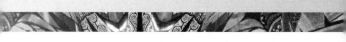

Contents

UNIT 4 DOCUMENTATION AND EVALUATION

UNIT 5 QUICK REFERENCE

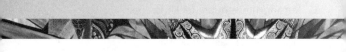

PREFACE

The *Clinical Handbook for Kozier & Erb's Fundamentals of Nursing*, 8e serves as a resource for students in the clinical area. It provides succinct information to guide you as you begin this important, exciting, and challenging component of your nursing program.

To keep this practical guide compact and portable, we have summarized key information designed to reinforce content that first must be learned thoroughly and carefully from *Fundamentals of Nursing*. The *Clinical Handbook* is not intended in any way to replace the text; rather, its purpose is to help you recall key points as you prepare to deliver safe and effective nursing care in a dynamic clinical environment. Before proceeding with the suggested guidelines and actions given in this book, check to determine an agency's policies, practices, and protocols.

The *Clinical Handbook* opens with a fundamental nursing unit that introduces the nursing process, delegation principles, and communication guidelines. Unit 2 reviews the processes for conducting a health history and physical examination. A complete list of the current North American Nursing Diagnosis Association (NANDA) nursing diagnoses is included. In Unit 3, we provide summaries of clinically related topics that you can expect to encounter routinely. Unit 4 presents documentation and evaluation principles. The handbook ends with a quick reference unit that presents essential information you will be able to retrieve rapidly. As you gain expertise in the clinical area, we believe you will continue to consult the *Clinical Handbook* again and again.

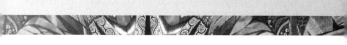

INTRODUCTION

On the first day of my pediatrics rotation, one of the children assigned to me was a 6-year-old asthmatic previously hospitalized several times for this same problem. Walking into his room with my instructor, I put forth what I thought was an air of confidence, even though my heart was beating a mile a minute. After the introductions, my little client reached for my hand and, with a voice of authority, told me not to be nervous, because he would tell me what I was supposed to do. Even though I was a little embarrassed that my cover was blown by a 6-year-old, I had to chuckle at being comforted by the client I was supposed to make comfortable. Welcome to the world of clinical rotations!

Clinical rotations give the student the opportunity to translate classroom theory and laboratory skills into action. This necessary and exciting part of nursing education, however, is often accompanied by feelings of apprehension and awkwardness. New situations heighten these feelings, as does the realization that you are still in transition between learning a skill and knowing how to use it efficiently. However, by being organized, being an active learner, and being good to yourself, you can use these feelings to challenge yourself and turn your clinical experiences into fun learning experiences.

Nursing is undergoing a wonderful evolution, and as a student, you bring to the process fresh views. The clients you will care for, the staff you will work with, and the facts you will learn about yourself will all help shape your views and turn you into the effective professional you want to be. No matter how difficult your day is, you should look on it as a learning experience. These difficult days give you precious knowledge that will make future days go easier. The following are tips to help you avoid some of the pitfalls that make the clinical experience unnecessarily stressful.

ORGANIZE

Clinical days always bring a little apprehension. Even as a senior, when the routines were familiar and the knowledge base was more solid, I still asked myself: "What will my instructor ask me? What emergencies will upset the schedule I set for myself? What if I oversleep and I'm late?"

To help combat this apprehension, I always reminded myself that there was nothing routine about client care, even though people talked about "hospital routines." There are only two predictable actions in nursing: (1) Clients will be cared for, and (2) documentation must be done. Everything else is subject to change!

To maintain your cool, do your work efficiently, and feel satisfied at the end of the day, you must be organized, set priorities, and remain flexible. Even if nothing else in your life is organized, be organized in your approach to the clinical experience. Remember also that organization and the ability to set priorities are behaviors instructors look for and grade on. The following are suggestions to help you become better organized:

- Arrive early. Set your alarm clock so that you arrive at the clinical site at least 20 minutes early. This gives you time to review the charts for any changes in doctor's orders, any orders that may have expired, or any tests that require your client to leave the floor. Doing this applies even if you cared for the same client the day before. Building in extra time also helps you on days when traffic is heavy or when you hit the snooze button once too often. The clinical experience can be stressful, so manage the stressors that are self-induced.

- Make a worksheet for reviewing charts. Include the name of the client, room number, diagnosis, primary nurse, times to assess vital signs, times to administer medications, equipment needs, procedures, and a space for comments. By making a note of the equipment you need, you can minimize the number of trips to the supply room (e.g., for dressing changes). Write in red all procedures or medications that are time sensitive. In addition to helping you organize your information, this also facilitates note writing and reporting to the primary nurse. On page xii is an example of a completed worksheet. See page xiii for a blank sample worksheet you can use.

- If possible, check the client's medications when you get to the unit. In some cases, medications are stored in secured cabinets, and students may not be permitted independent access to the keys or electronic codes. One of the most stressful situations you can face is to find yourself running late because of an intervening emergency, only to discover that the client's medications are not on the unit; meanwhile, your instructor is waiting for you to give the medications. By checking the Medication Administration Record, you can prepare yourself for this situation. If an order has expired, notify the primary nurse or the physician promptly, and note the fact on the chart. This shows your professionalism and, more important, gives you control of the situation.

- Attend report and/or talk to the primary nurse before you start. As a student, you must act as independently as possible in assessments and decision making; however, the primary nurse has ultimate responsibility for the client's care. In particular, find out about special circumstances relating to the client. For example, the primary nurse may tell you that the client does not eat breakfast until his wife arrives at 8:30 A.M. If this is not written in the chart, you may get yourself into a conflict with the client and learn about his preference the hard way. Knowing the details ahead of time can make your day easier.

Client's Initials/Rm # Diagnosis Primary RN	Vital Signs Blood Sugars	Medication Times	IVs Catheters I & O	Treatments Procedures	Comments
M.K. #323 DKA Ms. Wallace RN	V.S. qs B.S. 8 am 67 12 pm B.S.	8 am √ 12 pm √ 2 pm Colace refused	IVs-none Caths-none I&O-strict	None	O.J. Given at 8 am No insulin given this shift
M.B. #325 PUD Ms. Davies RN	V.S. q4 B.S. n/a	10 am √ 12 pm √ 2 pm √	IV-D5$^1/_2$NS@125/hr CATH-Foley I&O-none	UGI at 11 am Heme all stools Hep Flush q	NPO Client asked for communion this pm (called)

Client's Initials/Rm # Diagnosis Primary RN	Vital Signs Blood Sugars	Medication Times	IVs Catheters I & O	Treatments Procedures	Comments

- Do an "eyeball assessment" of each client's room before you start your day. Introduce yourself to the client and then look at whatever equipment is in the room. (Do not examine the client; you will do that when your shift begins.) Is there an IV? Is it dated and timed? Is it about to run out? Is there a catheter? Is the client being tube-fed? You will go over this information in the report, but having it beforehand can help make you a more active participant.

On your first day in a new unit or hospital, you will receive an orientation to the unit. After this orientation, do your own inspection and find out how the supply room is organized—for example, where the 4×4 gauzes, catheter setups, and so on, are located. Review fire exits and where emergency equipment such as the "code" cart and fire extinguishers are located. Also, find out where the staff bathroom is! When you get busy, it is nice to be able to save steps.

By staying organized and taking control of those things that you can, you can minimize stress and develop good habits that will stay with you throughout your career.

LEARN BEYOND THE HERE AND NOW

Nursing practice is based on understanding how to integrate knowledge from many sources and how to translate theory and facts into action. Clinical rotations offer a wonderful opportunity to do this, but keep in mind that you need to focus primarily on how to help the client and not on how to get a good grade. Sometimes, the pressure to perform well for a good grade gets in the way of the learning experience. However, if you focus on the needs of your client, a good grade will follow. As a nursing student, you have many ways to learn about nursing while still placing highest priority on your client's needs. Review all pathophysiology and nursing theory related to your client's diagnosis, no matter how confident you feel about your knowledge base. After reviewing the pathophysiology, jot down the laboratory studies, procedures, and medications you would expect to find ordered on the chart.

Also jot down signs and symptoms you would expect to see in the client. Compare your list to what actually appears in the chart. Compare your physical assessment findings with what you put on your list. How do the lists differ? How are they the same? Do not let your title, "nursing student," prevent you from being an active member of the health care team.

Ask questions of and talk with your instructor, other nurses, and other members of the health care team. Remember, the only dumb question is the one not asked. Read journal articles that relate to your clients' diagnoses.

Almost all hospitals have a library with current journals. After you leave the unit, make it a point to look for a new article that pertains to at least one of your clients. Imagine the pleasure of being able to answer an instructor's question about a client's course of treatment with, "A study reported in the latest issue of *Nursing Research* found that...." This not only makes a positive impression, but also helps you learn. Although it may be tough to fit into your schedule, reading journals should become a habit.

TAKE CARE OF YOURSELF

Above all else, take care of yourself. There is no way to give good client care if you cannot concentrate because you are hungry or frazzled. The following are suggestions for minimizing some of life's irritations that can interfere with the business of learning nursing:

- Eat a good meal before clinical rotations. It may sound trite, but given the unpredictability of the hospital day, you cannot always depend on having time for a break.

- Organize your things the day before.

- If you drive, make sure the car has gas. There is nothing worse than realizing that your tank is empty, and all the gas stations are closed.

- Keep some raisins or your favorite energy booster in your pocket for a quick pickup.

- If you are feeling harried, stop for a minute, and take a deep breath or two.

- Do not ever be afraid to ask for help.

- Keep a sense of humor.

Like anything else, the process of learning nursing can be frightening at first. The idea of practicing on real clients can be disconcerting. However, with some forethought and assertiveness, you can make the process fun, challenging, and a source of wonderful anecdotes to tell for years to come.

Best wishes for a great career in nursing.

Merilyn D. Francis, BSN, RN
1994 Graduate, University of the District of Columbia

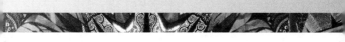

REVIEWERS

We would like to sincerely thank our student reviewers for their thoughtful feedback and suggestions.

Julie Bauder
Johns Hopkins University School of Nursing
Baltimore, Maryland

Marla Greco, BSN
The Pennsylvania State University
University Park, Pennsylvania

Melissa Whitty
The College of New Jersey
Ewing, New Jersey

FUNDAMENTAL NURSING

A. Components of the Nursing Process
B. Aspects of Delegation
C. Communication Guidelines

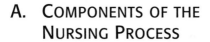

A. COMPONENTS OF THE NURSING PROCESS

The nursing process is a systematic, rational method of planning and providing individualized nursing care. Its goal is to identify a client's health status and actual or potential health care problems, to establish plans to meet the identified needs, and to deliver specific nursing interventions to meet those needs. The nursing process is cyclical; that is, the components of the nursing process follow a logical sequence, but more than one component may be involved at any one time. The five components of the nursing process are the following:

1. *Assessing*—collecting, organizing, validating, and documenting data about a client's health status to establish a database. Activities include obtaining a health history, performing a physical assessment, reviewing client records, reviewing literature, and consulting support people and health professionals.

2. *Diagnosing*—the process of analyzing and synthesizing data, which results in a diagnostic statement or nursing diagnosis. Activities include clustering data; comparing data against standards; generating tentative hypotheses; identifying gaps and inconsistencies; determining the client's health strengths, risks, and problems; and formulating nursing diagnosis statements.

3. *Planning*—a series of steps in which the nurse and the client set priorities, goals, or desired outcomes and establish a written care plan designed to resolve

or minimize the identified problems of the client and to coordinate the care provided by all health team members. Activities include setting priorities with the client, writing evaluation goals and outcome criteria with the client, selecting nursing interventions, consulting with other health care personnel, writing nursing interventions and nursing care plans, and communicating the care plan to relevant health care providers.

4. *Implementing*—putting the nursing care plan into action to help the client attain goals. Activities include reassessing the client, updating the database, reviewing and revising the care plan, and performing or delegating planned nursing interventions.

5. *Evaluating*—measuring the degree to which goals/ outcomes have been achieved and identifying factors that promote or impede goal achievement. Activities include collecting data about the client's response, comparing the client's response to evaluation criteria, relating nursing actions to client outcomes, making decisions about problem status, and modifying the care plan.

Refer to Chapters 10–14 of *Fundamentals of Nursing* for a thorough discussion of the components of the nursing process.

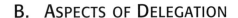

B. Aspects of Delegation

In nursing, delegation refers to indirect care—the intended outcome is achieved through the work of someone supervised by the nurse—and involves defining the task, determining who can perform the task, describing the expectation, seeking agreement, monitoring performance, and providing feedback to the delegate regarding performance. The National Council of State Boards of Nursing published five "rights" of delegation: The nurse delegates the *right task,* under the *right circumstances,* to the *right person,* with the *right direction and communication,* and the *right supervision and evaluation* (National Council of State Boards of Nursing, 1995). Once the decision has been made to delegate, the nurse must communicate clearly and verify that the person understands the following:

- The specific tasks to be done for each client
- When each task is to be done
- The expected outcomes for each task including parameters outside of which an unlicensed person must immediately report to the nurse (and any action that must urgently be taken)
- Who is available to serve as a resource if needed
- When and in what format (written or verbal) a report on the tasks is expected

See Table 1–1 for examples of tasks that may and may not be delegated to unlicensed assistive personnel.

Table 1–1   Examples of Tasks That May and May Not Be Delegated to Unlicensed Assistive Personnel

Tasks That *May* Be Delegated to Unlicensed Assistive Personnel	Tasks That *May Not* Be Delegated to Unlicensed Assistive Personnel
• Taking vital signs	• Assessment
• Measuring and recording intake and output	• Interpretation of data
• Client transfers and ambulation	• Nursing diagnosis
• Postmortem care	• Creation of a nursing care plan
• Bathing	• Evaluation of care effectiveness
• Feeding	• Care of invasive lines
• Gastrostomy feedings in established systems	• Administering parenteral medications
• Safety measures	• Venipuncture
• Weighing	• Insertion of nasogastric tubes
• Simple dressing changes	• Client education
• Suction of chronic tracheostomies	• Triage
• Basic life support (cardio-pulmonary resuscitation)	• Telephone advice

Principles Used by the Nurse to Determine Delegation to Unlicensed Assistive Personnel

1. The nurse must assess the individual client prior to delegating tasks.

2. The client must be medically stable or in a chronic condition and not fragile.

3. The task must be considered routine for this client.

4. The task must not require a substantial amount of scientific knowledge or technical skill.

5. The task must be considered safe for this client.

6. The task must have a predictable outcome.

7. Learn the agency's procedures and policies about delegation.

8. Know the scope of practice and the customary knowledge, skills, and job description for each health care discipline represented on your team.

9. Be aware of individual variations in work abilities. Along with different categories of caregivers are individual variations. Each individual has different experiences and may not be capable of performing every task cited in the job description.

10. When unsure about an assistant's abilities to perform a task, observe while the person performs it, or demonstrate it to the person and get a return demonstration before allowing the person to perform it independently.

11. Clarify reporting expectations to ensure the task is accomplished.

12. Create an atmosphere that fosters communication, teaching, and learning. For example, encourage staff to ask questions, listen carefully to their concerns, and make use of every opportunity to teach.

References

National Council of State Boards of Nursing. (1995). *Delegation: Concepts and decision-making process*. Chicago: Author.

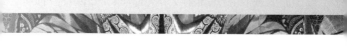

C. Communication Guidelines

Communication is a vital part of nursing practice. Nurses who communicate effectively are better able to initiate change that promotes health; establish a trusting relationship with clients, families, and colleagues; and prevent legal problems associated with nursing practice. Interpersonal attitudes are important. They convey beliefs, thoughts, and feelings about people and events. Attitudes such as caring, warmth, respect, and acceptance facilitate communication, whereas condescension, lack of interest, and coldness inhibit communication. Effective communication is essential to establishing a positive nurse–client relationship. Refer to Chapter 26 of *Fundamentals of Nursing* for a thorough discussion of communication techniques.

Therapeutic communication techniques can help promote understanding between nurse and client. These techniques include the following:

- Being silent when appropriate
- Asking open-ended questions
- Using touch when appropriate
- Restating or paraphrasing
- Seeking clarification
- Summarizing

In some situations, ordinary methods of communication are not sufficient: for example, when caring for a client who is angry, is confused, or speaks a language foreign to you. Some cultural issues also require sensitivity and understanding.

The Angry Client

Anger can be the result of fear, frustration, or a feeling of losing control. Often clients direct their anger toward the nurse, simply because the nurse is there. Angry outbursts from clients may be due to worries about their job, family, or illness. Fatigue or physical discomfort can also provoke anger. It is important that you try to identify the cause of the anger and not to feed that anger; maintain your composure.

The following are guidelines for responding to the angry client:

- Listen to what the client is saying.
- Do not let the client's anger cause you to react and not listen.
- Use techniques such as reflection, clarification, and focusing to determine the problem. Only when you understand the problem can you formulate a plan for resolution.
- Once the problem is identified, find ways to resolve it. Remember, **do not make promises you cannot keep.** A trusting relationship is key in diffusing angry outbursts.
- If you cannot resolve the client's anger, or if you feel any threat of violence, ask your instructor or the primary nurse for assistance.
- Be sure to document the conversation or incident, no matter how minor it may seem.

The Confused Client

Confusion in a client can be caused by medications, disease process, or the disruption of circadian rhythms. Whatever the cause, working with the confused client can be frustrating, so it is important to know your trigger points and what soothes them.

The following are guidelines for responding to the confused client:

- If this confusion is a new occurrence, review the client's medications and the potential side effects. Sudden onset of confusion is a sign that *must* be reported. Review your findings with your instructor.

- At every interaction with the client, orient the client to person, time, and place. Try to interact with the client as often as possible.

- Actively listen to the client, and clarify any points of confusion. Be attentive.

- Ask the family to orient the client as well. Be sensitive to the family's needs; they too can become frustrated.

- Reassure the client, but do not be condescending.

The Anxious Client

Fear of the unknown causes anxiety. All of us experience it at one time or another. As a nurse, it is important that you identify the causes or origin of a client's fear or anxiety.

The following are guidelines to use in responding to the anxious client:

- Talk to the client and actively listen. Answer all questions you can answer accurately. Use the skills of reflection, clarification, and focusing to get the client to talk about the true problem.

- Questions such as "Am I going to die?" or "Do I have AIDS or cancer?" are the most disconcerting. Ask clients what makes them believe that they are going to die or that they have acquired immunodeficiency syndrome or cancer. Your goal is to get them to verbalize their fears.

- If the client has questions about the medical diagnosis, find out what the client has already been told. Clarify any points you can. If the client has not been told anything, ask whether the client would like to speak to the primary care provider. It is the primary care provider's responsibility, not yours, to communicate the diagnosis.

- Be attentive to the client. Check in on the client as much as possible. This establishes trust and communicates a caring attitude.

- Above all, do not be condescending or dismiss the client's anxiety. Put yourself in the client's position.

Communicating Across Language Barriers

There are many types of language barriers. Foreign language, hearing deficits, expressive disorders (e.g., aphasia), and intubation are all barriers to effective communication and require some creativity, patience, and perseverance. It is crucial for the client to be able to communicate needs and for the nurse to be able to communicate understanding. Health care facilities usually have resources that can help you, such as translation services for the non–English-speaking client and for the hearing-impaired. The speech therapy department can help you find ways to communicate with a client who has speech deficits.

The Non–English-Speaking Client

- Find out whether the health care facility has a translation service.

- Find out if any staff members speak the language.

- Do not yell at the client. Speaking more loudly may only make the client think you are angry. If the client does not understand English, increasing the decibel level does not help.

- If a particular language is commonly spoken at the facility (e.g., Spanish), purchase a phrase book and take the opportunity to add to your skills. You may also wish to develop a resource binder containing frequently used terms in many languages.

- If all else fails, act out what you are going to do. This does work.

- As a last resort, enlist the help of a family member or friend who may be able to translate. However, be considerate of these people; translating can be very stressful. Remember that they are the client's support system, not yours. Also, clients may be reluctant to share intimate health information with family members.

The Hearing-Impaired Client

- Stand in front of the hearing-impaired client and talk distinctly at a normal tone. Make sure the client can clearly see you. Many clients who are hard-of-hearing read lips.

- Keep paper and pencil at the bedside and write notes, especially when privacy is important.

- For the client who uses sign language, enlist the help of a translation service, if available.

- If no services are available to help you and writing is not possible, act out what you would like to do.

- Take the opportunity to learn sign language.

The Client with Aphasia

- Listen carefully. Encourage clients to take their time. Do not be afraid to ask clients to repeat themselves.

- Use paper and pencil, or picture board, if appropriate.

- If the aphasia is a long-standing condition, ask a family member for assistance.

- Call the speech therapy department for any additional help, if needed.

The Intubated Client

- Use paper and pencil for communication or a letter board on which the client can spell out words.

- If yes-or-no answers are needed, have the client blink once for yes and twice for no.

Cultural Issues

In almost every area of the country, nurses come into contact with people from cultures different from their own. Although it is not within the scope of this book to describe the differences in all cultures you may encounter, some universal guidelines can be of help.

Examine your own attitudes. What are your attitudes toward different cultures? What experiences have you had with different races and ethnic groups? What influences your acceptance or nonacceptance of a cultural group? Are your beliefs about a certain culture based on experience or on what you have heard or read? Refer to Chapter 18 of *Fundamentals of Nursing* for a thorough discussion of cultural issues.

The following are guidelines for responding to clients of different cultures:

- Always treat the client with respect.

- Different cultures may use different behaviors to denote respect or understanding. Do not assume you know the meaning of a specific behavior.

- Familiarize yourself with the customs and beliefs of cultural groups in your area.

- Try to incorporate cultural symbols and practices into the care plan of the client where feasible; these can bring comfort to a client.

- Remember that the color of a person's skin does not necessarily indicate the person's cultural background.

- Learn how the client views health, illness, grieving, and the health care system.

Special Care for Elders

Communication

It is important that health care providers who work with elders increase their awareness of and avoid the use of *elderspeak*. Elderspeak is a speech style similar to baby talk. It does not communicate respect, but instead gives the message of dependence and incompetence to older adults. The characteristics of elderspeak include the following:

- Inappropriate terms of endearment (e.g., honey, sweetie)

- Inappropriate plural nouns (e.g., "Are *we* ready for *our* medicine?)

- Tag questions that prompt the answer and imply that the elder cannot act alone (e.g., "You would rather wear the blue shirt, *wouldn't you*?")

- Baby talk instead of the usual sentence structure, speech rate, and vocabulary

Elders may have physical or cognitive problems that necessitate nursing interventions for improvement of communication skills. Some of the common ones are the following:

- Sensory deficits, such as vision and hearing
- Cognitive impairment, as in dementia
- Neurologic deficits from strokes or other neurologic conditions, such as aphasia (expressive and/or receptive) and lack of movement
- Psychosocial problems, such as depression

Recognizing specific needs and obtaining appropriate resources for clients can greatly increase their socialization and quality of life. Interventions directed toward improving communication in clients with these special needs are the following:

- Ensuring that assistive devices, glasses, and hearing aids are being used and are in good working order
- Making referrals to appropriate resources, such as speech therapy
- Making use of communications aids, such as communication boards, computers, and pictures, when possible
- Keeping environmental distractions to a minimum
- Speaking in short, simple sentences, one subject at a time—reinforce or repeat what is said when necessary
- Always facing the person when speaking—coming up behind someone may be frightening
- Including family and friends in conversation
- Using reminiscing, either in individual conversations or in groups to maintain memory connections and to enhance self-identity and self-esteem in the elder
- Believing the nonverbal when verbal expression and nonverbal expression are incongruent (Clarification of this and attentiveness to the elder's feelings help promote a feeling of caring and acceptance.)
- Finding out what has been important and has meaning to the person and trying to maintain these things as much as possible (Even simple things such as bed-

time rituals become important if he or she is lost in a hospital or extended-care setting.)

Communication Among Health Professionals

Effective communication among the health professions is as important as the promotion of therapeutic communication between the nurse and the client. Skilled communication is critical for a number of situations: preserving a nurse's professional integrity while ensuring a client's safety, during nurse and physician communication, and at change-of-shift reporting.

Nurses need to be as proficient in communication skills as they are in clinical skills. The American Association of Critical-Care Nurses developed standards for establishing and sustaining health work environments. The association's communication standard includes the following critical elements for the nurse (American Association of Critical-Care Nurses, 2005):

- Skilled communicators focus on finding solutions and achieving desirable outcomes.

- Skilled communicators seek to protect and advance collaborative relationships among colleagues.

- Skilled communicators invite and hear all relevant perspectives.

- Skilled communicators call upon goodwill and mutual respect to build consensus and arrive at common understanding.

- Skilled communicators demonstrate congruence between words and actions, holding others accountable for doing the same.

- Skilled communicators have access to appropriate communications technologies and are proficient in their use.

Few guidelines exist for the frequent verbal communication that occurs between nurses and doctors. One model, called the *situational briefing model*, provides a framework for nurses when communicating with a physician.

A FRAMEWORK FOR NURSE–PHYSICIAN COMMUNICATION
Provide the following:
- Information about the client's current situation
- Background for the current clinical situation
- Assessment of the current problem
- Recommendation that addresses the client's need

Note: From "Improving Verbal Communication in Clinical Care" by S. **Beyea**, 2004, *AORN Journal, 79*(5), 1053–1057.

A change-of-shift report is given to all nurses on the next shift. It communicates a quick summary of client needs and details of care to be given for the new caregivers. Key elements of a change-of-shift report include the following:

Box 1-2 Key Elements of Change-of-Shift Report

- Follow a particular order (e.g., follow room numbers in a hospital).
- Provide basic identifying information for each client (e.g., name, room number, bed designation).
- For new clients, provide the reason for admission or medical diagnosis (or diagnoses), surgery (date), diagnostic tests, and therapies in past 24 hours.
- Include significant changes in client's condition and present information in order (i.e., assessment, nursing diagnoses, interventions, outcomes, and evaluation). For example, "Mr. Ronald Oakes said he had an aching pain in his left calf at 1400 hours. Inspection revealed no other signs. Calf pain is related to altered blood circulation. Rest and elevation of his legs on a footstool for 30 minutes provided relief."
- Provide exact information, such as "Ms. Jessie Jones received morphine, 6 mg IV at 1500 hours," not "Ms. Jessie Jones received some morphine during the evening."

- Report client's need for special emotional support. For example, a client who has just learned that his biopsy results revealed a malignancy and who is now scheduled for a laryngectomy needs time to discuss his feelings before preoperative teaching is begun.
- Include current nurse-prescribed and primary care provider–prescribed orders.
- Provide a summary of newly admitted clients, including diagnosis, age, general condition, plan of therapy, and significant information about the client's support people.
- Report on clients who have been transferred or discharged from the unit.
- Clearly state priorities of care and care that is due after the shift begins. For example, in a 7 a.m. report, the nurse might say, "Mr. Li's vital signs are due at 0730, and his IV bag will need to be replaced by 0800." Give this information at the end of that client's report because memory is best for the first and last information given.
- Be concise. Don't elaborate on background data or routine care (e.g., do not report "vital signs at 0800 and 1150" when that is the unit standard). Do not report coming and going of visitors unless there is a problem or concern, or visitors are involved in teaching and care. Social support and visits are the norm.

References

American Association of Critical-Care Nurses. (2005). *AACN standards for establishing and sustaining healthy work environments: A journey to excellence.* Aliso Viejo, CA: Author.

ASSESSMENT AND DIAGNOSIS

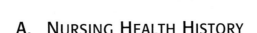

A. Nursing Health History

The nursing health history is the first part of the assessment of the client's health status. Through this structured interview, you collect specific health data and obtain a detailed health record of the client. The client is the primary source of information.

You may also consult other sources for information about the client's health, including the medical record if available, and consultations with members of the health care team, family members, or significant others. It is important to be systematic in your approach and document your findings.

Before starting the interview, be sure to introduce yourself and state your purpose for collecting data. Establish rapport to put the client at ease and facilitate the interview process.

Biographic Data
- Obtain client's name, address, age, sex, marital status, occupation, religious preference, health care financing, and usual source of medical care.

Chief Complaint or Reason for Visit
- The answer given to the question "What is troubling you?" or "What brought you to the hospital or clinic?" is the chief complaint, which should be recorded in the client's own words.

History of Present Illness
- When the symptoms started
- Whether the onset of symptoms was sudden or gradual
- How often the problem occurs

- Exact location of the distress
- Character of the complaint (e.g., intensity of pain or quality of sputum, emesis, or discharge)
- Activity in which the client was involved when the problem occurred
- Phenomena or symptoms associated with the chief complaint
- Factors that aggravate or alleviate the problem

Past History

- Childhood illnesses, such as chickenpox, mumps, measles, rubella (German measles), rubeola (red measles), streptococcal infections, scarlet fever, rheumatic fever, and other significant illnesses
- Childhood immunizations and date of the last tetanus shot
- Allergies to foods, drugs, animals, insects, or other environmental agents and the type of reaction that occurs
- Injuries: how, when, and where the incident occurred; type of injury; treatment received; and any complications
- Acute or chronic diseases, such as asthma, high blood pressure, cancer, seizures, diabetes, arthritis, stroke, hepatitis, human immunodeficiency virus
- Hospitalization for serious illnesses: reasons for the hospitalization, dates, surgery performed, course of recovery, and any complications
- Medications: all currently used prescription and over-the-counter medications, such as aspirin, nasal spray, vitamins, or laxatives; herbs; and homeopathic remedies

Family History of Illness

- Ages of siblings, parents, and grandparents and their current state of health or the cause of death (if they are deceased); particular attention to disorders such as heart disease, cancer, diabetes, hypertension, obesity, allergies, arthritis, tuberculosis, bleeding, alcoholism, and any mental health disorders

Lifestyle

- Personal habits: the amount, frequency, and duration of substance use (tobacco, alcohol, coffee, cola, tea, and illicit or recreational drugs)
- Diet: description of a typical diet on a normal day or any special diet, number of meals and snacks per day, who cooks and shops for food, ethnically distinct food patterns, and allergies
- Sleep/rest patterns: usual daily sleep/wake times, difficulties sleeping, and remedies used for difficulties
- Activities of daily living: any difficulties experienced in the basic activities of eating, grooming, dressing, elimination, and locomotion
- Recreation/hobbies: exercise activity and tolerance, hobbies and other interests, and vacations

Social Data

- Family relationships/friendships: the client's support system (those who help in time of need), effect the client's illness has on the family, whether any family problems are affecting the client
- Ethnic affiliation: health customs and beliefs; cultural practices that may affect health care and recovery
- Educational history: data about the client's highest level of education attained and any past difficulties with learning
- Occupational history: current employment status, days missed from work because of illness, history of accidents on the job, occupational hazards with a potential for future disease or accident, client's need to change jobs because of past illness, employment status of spouses or partners and the way child care is handled, and client's overall satisfaction with work
- Economic status: how the client pays for medical care (including what kind of medical and hospitalization coverage the client has) and whether the client's illness presents financial concerns

- Home and neighborhood conditions: home safety measures and adjustments in physical facilities that may be required to help the client manage physical disability, activity intolerance, and activities of daily living; availability of neighborhood and community services to meet the client's needs

Psychological Data

- Major stressors experienced and the client's perception of them
- Usual coping pattern with a serious problem or a high level of stress
- Communication style: ability to verbalize appropriate emotion; nonverbal communication such as eye movements, gestures, use of touch, and posture; interactions with support persons; and congruence of nonverbal behavior and verbal expression

Patterns of Health Care

- Health care resources the client is currently using and has used in the past (e.g., family physician, specialists such as ophthalmologist or gynecologist, dentist, folk practitioners, health clinic, or health center); whether the client considers the care being provided adequate; and whether access to health care is a problem

Review of Systems

The goal of the review of systems is to gather subjective data from the client on each of the major body systems.

- *General health.* Weight loss, weakness, feelings of fatigue, mood changes, night sweats, or bleeding tendencies?
- *Skin.* Skin diseases such as eczema, psoriasis, acne; change in pigmentation; tendency toward bruising; excessive dryness or moisture; jaundice; itching, rashes, hives; change in color or size of moles; or open sores that are slow to heal?
- *Hair.* Itchy scalp, loss of hair, excessive body hair? Does the client wear a wig?

- *Nails.* Color changes, biting, clubbing, splitting?
- *Head.* Frequent or severe headaches, fainting, dizziness, accident resulting in unconsciousness?
- *Eyes.* Difficulty seeing, eye infection, eye pain, excessive tearing, double vision, blurring, sensitivity to light, cataracts, itching, spots in front of eyes? Does the client wear glasses (for near or far vision) or contact lenses? When was the client's last eye examination?
- *Ears.* Any infection, loss of hearing, pain, discharge, ringing in the ears? Does the client wear a hearing aid?
- *Nose.* Frequent colds, nosebleeds, allergies, pain, tenderness, postnasal drip?
- *Mouth and throat.* Sore gums; bleeding gums; sores, lumps or white spots on mouth, lips, or tongue; toothaches, cavities, or difficulty swallowing; voice change or hoarseness? Does the client wear dentures (upper, lower, partial)? When was the client's last dental appointment?
- *Neck.* Pain, swelling, stiffness, limited movement, swollen glands?
- *Breasts.* Nipple discharge, scaling or cracks around nipples, dimples, lumps, pattern of breast self-examination? Last mammogram?
- *Respiratory system.* Chest pain; cough; shortness of breath; wheezing; coughing up blood; lung disease such as tuberculosis, emphysema, asthma, or bronchitis? Has the client ever had a chest x-ray? When? Results?
- *Cardiovascular system.* Heart disease, palpitations, heart murmur, high blood pressure, anemia, varicose veins, leg swelling or ulcer?
- *Gastrointestinal system.* Nausea, vomiting, loss of appetite, indigestion, heartburn, bright blood in stools, tarry-black stools, diarrhea, constipation, abdominal pain, excessive gas, hemorrhoids, rectal pain, colostomy, ileostomy?

- *Genitourinary system.* Frequency, dribbling, urgency, urination at night, difficulty starting stream, blood in urine, incontinence, pain or burning upon urination, urinary tract infection, ureterostomy, sexually transmitted disease such as gonorrhea or syphilis?
  - *Females*: Age of menarche, last menstrual period, duration, amount of flow, regularity of cycle? Any problems with painful menstruation, bleeding between periods, pain during intercourse, vaginal discharge, vaginal itching, vaginal infection?
  - *Males*: Penile discharge, swelling, masses or lesions, difficulty in sexual functioning?
- *Musculoskeletal system.* Muscular pain, swelling, or weakness; joint swelling, soreness, or stiffness; leg cramps; bone defects?
- *Neurologic system.* Difficulty walking; unconsciousness; seizures; tremors; paralysis; numbness, tingling, or burning sensations in any body part; weakness on one side of body; speech problems; loss of memory; disorientation; forgetfulness; unclear thinking; changes in emotional state?
- *Endocrine system.* History of goiter, heat or cold intolerance, diabetes, excessive thirst, excessive eating?

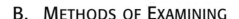

B. Methods of Examining

The four primary techniques used in the physical examination are inspection, palpation, percussion, and auscultation.

Inspection
Inspection, or visual examination, should be done systematically, with sufficient light.

Palpation
Palpation is the use of the sense of touch to determine texture, temperature, vibration, position, size, consistency, mobility, distention, pulse rates, and tenderness or pain.

Percussion
In percussion, the body surface is struck to elicit sounds that can be heard or vibrations that can be felt.

Percussion is used to determine the size and shape of the internal organs by establishing their borders. It indicates whether tissue is fluid-filled, air-filled, or solid. Percussion elicits five types of sounds:

- Flatness (dull)—bone and muscle
- Dullness (thudlike)—liver, spleen, heart
- Resonance (hollow)—air-filled lung
- Hyperresonance (booming)—emphysematous lung
- Tympany (drumlike)—air-filled stomach

The two types of percussion methods are direct/immediate and indirect/mediate.

Direct Percussion

- Strike the area to be percussed with two or more fingers, using the pads of the fingers only.
- Use rapid wrist movements.

Indirect Percussion

- Place the middle finger of your nondominant hand firmly on the skin of the area to be percussed. (Use only the distal phalanx and joint of the finger.)
- Using the flexed middle finger of the dominant hand, strike the middle finger of the nondominant hand. Be sure to use rapid wrist movements.

Auscultation

Auscultation is the process of listening to sounds produced within the body. The use of an unaided ear is the direct method of auscultation. The use of a stethoscope is considered an indirect method. Auscultated sounds are described according to the following:

- Pitch—frequency of vibrations
- Intensity—loudness or softness
- Duration—length of the sound
- Quality—subjective description of the sound

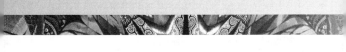

C. VITAL SIGNS

Vital signs are obtained to monitor the functions of the body. The temperature, pulse, respiratory rate, blood pressure, and oxygen concentration measurements indicate how the body is functioning or responding to medications or treatments. Refer to Chapter 29 of *Fundamentals of Nursing* for a thorough discussion of vital signs. Many people consider pain to be one of the vital signs. See Unit 3, Clinical Guidelines 2, for details on pain assessment and treatment.

Temperature

Temperature is a measurement of the balance between heat produced by the body and heat lost from the body. A fever results from inadequate heat loss; a low temperature results from excessive heat loss. When measured orally, adult temperature is 36.7°C to 37°C. Leave the thermometer in place for the length of time recommended for the type of thermometer and location of measurement. Temperatures can be taken via the following methods:

- Oral—If the client is too young or too confused to cooperate, use another means of measuring temperature.
- Rectal—Use water-soluble lubricant to insert the thermometer. Do not use the rectal method if client has rectal disease or convulsions. Be sure to hold a child firmly.
- Axillary—Wipe the axillary area if damp. After placing the thermometer, hold the arm against the chest.

Pulse

The pulse is a wave of blood created by contraction of the heart's left ventricle. The nine sites where pulses are commonly taken are (1) temporal, (2) carotid, (3) apical, (4) brachial, (5) radial (most common), (6) femoral, (7) popliteal, (8) posterior tibial, and (9) pedal. See Figure 2–1 for pulse sites.

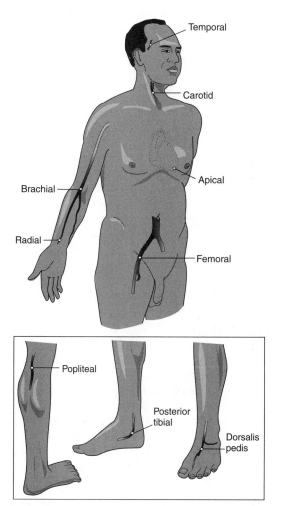

Figure 2–1 ■ Nine sites for taking pulses.

To take a client's pulse, proceed with the following steps:

- Before taking the pulse, ensure that the client is at rest. If the client has been active, wait 10 to 15 minutes.
- Use your index and middle fingers to palpate all pulse sites, except for the apex of the heart, where a stethoscope is required.
- Note rate, rhythm, volume, arterial wall elasticity, presence of bilateral equality, and intensity.
- Count irregular pulses a full 60 seconds.

Respirations

When assessing respirations, note the rate (breaths per minute), depth (normal, deep, or shallow), rhythm (regularity), and quality (effort required to breathe, and the sound of the respirations). When possible, use the following methods to assess respirations, when the client is unaware that you are doing so:

- While standing at the bedside, ask the client to place the arm farthest away from you across the chest, if possible. The arm will rise and fall as the client breathes, making it easier to count respirations.
- After assessing the pulse, continue holding the wrist. Count the respiratory rate and observe the depth, rhythm, and quality of respirations.

Blood Pressure

Blood pressure is a measure of the pressure the blood exerts as it flows through the arteries. The systolic pressure (the top number) measures the amount of pressure during contraction of the ventricles, and the diastolic pressure (the bottom number) is the measure of the pressure in the arteries when the ventricles are at rest. Blood pressures can be taken on the arm or on the thigh. Points to remember include the following:

- Be sure the cuff is of adequate size. For the obese client, use a large or thigh cuff. The cuff should be wide enough to cover two-thirds of the upper arm.
- Make sure the client is calm and has not smoked or exercised within 30 minutes of the measurement.

- Inspect the arm or thigh before placing the cuff. Do not use an extremity that has an IV line or is injured.

- Use the bell side of the amplifier of the stethoscope over the pulse site.

- Pump up the cuff until the sphygmomanometer reads 30 mm Hg above the point where the pulse disappeared.

- Release the valve on the cuff so that the pressure decreases at the rate of 2 to 3 mm Hg per second. Note the readings at Korotkoff phase 1 (first faint, clear tapping or thumping sounds), phase 4 (muffled and soft, blowing quality), and phase 5 (last sound is heard). Record as phase 1/phase 5 or phase 1/phase 4/phase 5, depending on agency policy.

- Wait 1 to 2 minutes before making further determinations.

- If this is the client's initial examination, repeat the procedure on the client's other arm.

Oxygen Saturation

A pulse oximeter is a noninvasive device that estimates a client's arterial blood oxygen saturation (SaO_2) by means of a sensor attached to the client's finger, toe, nose, earlobe, or forehead and reports a percent SpO_2.

- Choose a sensor appropriate for the client's weight, size, and desired location.

- If the client is allergic to adhesive, use a clip or sensor without adhesive. If using an extremity, assess the proximal pulse and capillary refill at the point closest to the site.

- Clean the site with an alcohol wipe before applying the sensor. It may be necessary to remove dark nail polish because it can interfere with accurate measurements or position the sensor on the side of the finger rather than perpendicular to the nail bed.

- Attach the sensor cable to the connection outlet on the oximeter (unless a wireless device is used).

- Ensure that the bar of light or waveform on the face of the oximeter fluctuates with each pulsation.

- When using continuous monitoring, check the alarm limits for high and low oxygen saturation and high and low pulse rates.

- Inspect the location of an adhesive toe or finger sensor every 4 hours and a spring-tension sensor every 2 hours.

- If indicated, cover the sensor with a sheet or towel to block large amounts of light from external sources (e.g., sunlight, procedure lamps, or bilirubin lights in the nursery).

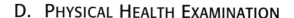

D. Physical Health Examination

A complete health assessment is generally conducted starting from the head and moving toward the toes; however, the procedure can vary in many ways according to the age of the individual, the severity of the illness, the preferences of the nurse, and the agency's priorities and procedures. Regardless of what procedure is used, the client's energy and time must be considered. The health assessment is therefore conducted in a systematic and efficient manner that requires the fewest position changes for the client.

Frequently, nurses assess a specific body area instead of the entire body. These specific assessments are made in relation to client complaints, the nurse's own observation of the problem, the client's presenting problem, nursing interventions provided, and medical therapies.

While you are assessing the client, do not be afraid to talk and ask questions. Conversation puts the client at ease and gives you valuable subjective information.

Preparing the Client

Most people need an explanation of the physical health examination. Explain when and where the examination will take place, why it is necessary, who will conduct it, and what will happen during the examination. Also inform the client of any special circumstances—for instance, the need to go to a different room or assume a special position—and tell the client that appropriate draping will be provided so that the body will not be unnecessarily exposed.

Most clients should empty the bladder before the examination. Doing so helps them feel more relaxed and facilitates palpation of the abdomen and pubic area. If a urinalysis is required, urine should be collected in a container for that purpose.

Before you start, be sure to do the following:

- Collect your equipment.
- Explain to the client what you will be doing and approximately how long it will take to complete the examination. Establishing rapport with the client makes for a more relaxed examination for both of you.
- Cleanse your hands. Follow infection control precautions throughout.
- Ensure that the client's privacy is protected. Draw the curtain if the room is semiprivate.

Assessing the Client
General Survey
Appearance

- Observe body build, height, and weight in relation to the client's age, lifestyle, and health.
- Observe the client's posture and gait, standing, sitting, and walking.
- Observe the client's overall hygiene and grooming. Relate these to the person's activities before the assessment.
- Note body and breath odor in relation to activity level.
- Observe for signs of distress in posture (e.g., bending over because of abdominal pain) or facial expressions (e.g., wincing or labored breathing).
- Note obvious signs of health or illness (e.g., in skin color or breathing).

Mental Status

- Assess the client's attitude.
- Note the client's affect/mood; assess the appropriateness of the client's responses.

- Listen for quantity of speech (amount and pace), quality (loudness, clarity, inflection), and organization (coherence of thought, overgeneralization, vagueness).
- Listen for relevance and organization of thoughts.

The Integument
Skin

- Inspect skin color (best assessed under natural lighting and on areas not exposed to the sun).
- Inspect uniformity of skin color.
- Assess edema if present (e.g., location, color, temperature, shape, and the number of millimeters to which the skin remains indented or pitted when pressed by a finger).
- Inspect, palpate, and describe skin lesions. Palpate lesions to determine shape and texture. Describe lesions according to location, distribution, color, configuration, size, shape, type, or structure.
- Observe and palpate skin moisture.
- Palpate skin temperature. Compare the two feet and two hands using the backs of your fingers.
- Note skin turgor (fullness or elasticity) by lifting and pinching the skin on an extremity.

Hair

- Inspect the distribution of growth over the scalp.
- Inspect hair thickness or thinness, texture, and oiliness.
- Note the presence of infections or infestations by parting the hair in several areas.
- Inspect amount of body hair.

Nails

- Inspect nail plate shape to determine its curvature and angle.
- Inspect nail texture.
- Inspect nail color.
- Inspect tissues surrounding nails.

- Perform blanch test to evaluate capillary refill.

The Head
The Skull and Face
- Inspect the skull for size, shape, and symmetry.
- Palpate the skull for masses, depressions, or nodules.
- Inspect the facial features (e.g., symmetry of structures).
- Inspect the eyes for edema and hollowness.
- Note symmetry of facial movements. Ask the client to elevate the eyebrows, frown or lower the eyebrows, close the eyes tightly, puff the cheeks, and smile and show teeth.

The Eyes and Vision
External Eye Structures
- Inspect the eyebrows for hair distribution, alignment, skin quality, and movement (ask the client to raise and lower the eyebrows).
- Inspect the eyelashes for evenness of distribution and direction of the curl.
- Inspect the eyelids for surface characteristics such as skin quality and texture, position in relation to the cornea, ability to blink, and frequency of blinking.
- Inspect the bulbar conjunctiva (the conjunctiva lying over the sclera) for color, texture, and presence of lesions. Retract the eyelids and ask client to look up, down, and from side to side.
- Inspect the palpebral conjunctiva (the conjunctiva lining the eyelids) by everting the lower lids. Note color, texture, and presence of lesions.
- Evert upper lids if a problem is suspected.
- Inspect and palpate the lacrimal gland, lacrimal sac, and nasolacrimal duct.
- Inspect the corneas for clarity and texture by using a penlight at an oblique angle to the eye.
- Perform corneal sensitivity (reflex) test to determine function of the fifth (trigeminal) cranial nerve.

- Inspect the anterior chamber for transparency and depth.
- Inspect pupils for color, shape, and symmetry of size.
- Assess each pupil's direct and consensual reaction to light to determine the function of the third (oculomotor) and fourth (trochlear) cranial nerves.
- Assess each pupil's reaction to accommodation.

Visual Fields

- Assess peripheral visual fields to determine function of the retina and neuronal visual pathways to the brain and second (optic) cranial nerve.

Extraocular Muscle Tests

- Assess six ocular movements to determine eye alignment and coordination.
- Perform the cover-uncover patch test to determine eye alignment.
- Perform the corneal light reflex test to determine eye alignment.

Visual Acuity

- Assess near vision by asking the client to wear corrective lenses if used for reading. Ask the client to read from a document held 36 cm (14 in.) from the face.
- Assess distance vision using the Snellen or similar chart (with the client wearing corrective lenses if required, unless they are used for reading only).
- Perform functional vision tests (e.g., light perception, hand movements, counting fingers at 1 foot) if the client is unable to see the top line of the Snellen chart.

The Ears and Hearing

Auricles

- Inspect the auricles for color, symmetry of size, and position.
- Palpate the auricles for texture, elasticity, and areas of tenderness.

External Ear Canal and Tympanic Membrane

- Using an otoscope, inspect the external ear canal for cerumen, skin lesions, pus, and blood. Inspect the tympanic membrane for color.

Gross Hearing Acuity Test

- Assess client's response to normal voice tones.
- Assess client's response to a whispered voice.

Tuning Fork Tests

- Perform Weber's test to assess bone conduction.
- Perform the Rinne test to compare air conduction to bone conduction.

Nose and Sinuses

- Inspect the external nose for any deviations in shape, size, symmetry, or color. Inspect for flaring or discharge from the nares.
- Lightly palpate the external nose to determine any areas of tenderness, masses, and displacements of bone and cartilage.
- Inspect the nasal cavities using a penlight or a nasal speculum.
- Determine patency of both nasal cavities.
- Palpate the maxillary and frontal sinuses for tenderness.
- Transilluminate the frontal and maxillary sinuses.

The Mouth and Oropharynx

Lips and Buccal Mucosa

- Inspect the outer lips for symmetry of contour, color, and texture.
- Inspect and palpate the inner lips and buccal mucosa for color, moisture, texture, and the presence of lesions.

Teeth and Gums

- Inspect the teeth and gums while examining the inner lips and buccal mucosa.
- Inspect the dentures. Ask the client to remove complete or partial dentures. Inspect their condition, noting in particular broken or worn areas.

Tongue/Floor of Mouth

- Inspect the surface of the tongue for position, color, and texture by asking the client to protrude the tongue.
- Inspect tongue movement.
- Inspect the base of the tongue, the mouth floor, and the frenulum.
- Palpate the tongue and floor of the mouth for any nodules, lumps, or excoriated areas.

Salivary Glands

- Inspect salivary gland openings for any swelling or redness.

Palates and Uvula

- Inspect the hard palate and soft palate for color, shape, texture, and the presence of bony prominences.
- Inspect the uvula for position and mobility while examining the palates.

Oropharynx and Tonsils

- Inspect the oropharynx for color and texture using a tongue blade and penlight.
- Inspect the tonsils for color, discharge, and size.
- Elicit the gag reflex by pressing the posterior tongue with a tongue depressor.

The Neck
Neck Muscles

- Inspect the neck muscles for abnormal swelling or masses.
- Observe head movement. Ask the client to move the chin to the chest, to move the head back so that the chin points upward, to move the head so that the ear is moved toward the shoulder on each side, and to turn the head to the right and to the left.
- Assess muscle strength by asking the client to turn the head against the resistance of your hand. Repeat with the other side. Then ask the client to shrug the shoulders against the resistance of your hands.

Lymph Nodes

- Palpate the entire neck for presence of enlarged lymph nodes.

Trachea

- Palpate the trachea for lateral deviation.

Thyroid Gland

- Inspect the thyroid gland by standing in front of the client.
- Observe the lower half of the neck overlying the thyroid gland for symmetry and visible masses.
- Ask the client to hyperextend the head and swallow to determine thyroid and cricoid movement.
- Palpate the thyroid gland for smoothness.
- If enlargement of the gland is suspected, auscultate over the thyroid area for a bruit.

The Thorax and Lungs
Posterior Thorax

- Inspect the shape and symmetry of the anterior, posterior, and lateral thorax.
- Inspect the spinal alignment for deformities.
- Palpate the posterior thorax.
- Palpate the posterior chest for respiratory excursion.
- Palpate the chest for vocal (tactile) fremitus, comparing each lung side.
- Percuss the thorax. Use a systematic zigzag procedure.
- Percuss for diaphragmatic excursion during maximal inspiration and expiration.
- Auscultate the chest using the flat-disc diaphragm of the stethoscope. Ask the client to take slow, deep breaths through the mouth. Use a systematic zigzag procedure. Compare findings at each point with the corresponding point on the opposite side of the chest. See Tables 2–1 and 2–2 for description of normal and adventitious breath sounds.

Table 2–1 Normal Breath Sounds

Type	Description	Location	Characteristics
Vesicular	Soft-intensity, low- pitched, "gentle sighing" sounds created by air moving through smaller airways (bronchioles and alveoli)	Over peripheral lung; best heard at base of lungs	Best heard on inspiration, which is about 2.5 times longer than the expiratory phase (5:2 ratio)
Broncho-vesicular	Moderate-intensity and moderate-pitched "blowing" sounds created by air moving through larger airway (bronchi)	Between the scapulae and lateral to the sternum at the first and second intercostal spaces	Equal inspiratory and expiratory phases (1:1 ratio)
Bronchial (tubular)	High-pitched, loud, "harsh" sounds created by air moving through the trachea	Anteriorly over the trachea; not normally heard over lung tissue	Louder than vesicular sounds; have a short inspiratory phase and long expiratory phase (1:2 ratio)

Anterior Thorax

- Inspect breathing patterns (e.g., respiratory rate and rhythm).

- Inspect the costal angle and the angle at which the ribs enter the spine.

- Palpate the anterior chest for respiratory excursion and tactile fremitus.

- Percuss the anterior chest symmetrically. Begin above the clavicles in the supraclavicular space, and proceed down to the diaphragm. Compare one side of the lung to the other.

- Auscultate the trachea.

- Auscultate the anterior chest. Use the sequence used in percussion, beginning over the bronchi between the ster-

Table 2–2 Adventitious Breath Sounds

Name	Description	Cause	Location
Crackles (rales)	Fine, short, interrupted crackling sounds; alveolar rales are high-pitched. Sound can be simulated by rolling a lock of hair near the ear. Best heard on inspiration but can be heard on both inspiration and expiration. May not be cleared by coughing	Air passing through fluid or mucus in any air passage	Most commonly heard in the bases of the lower lung lobes
Gurgles (rhonchi)	Continuous, low-pitched, coarse, gurgling, harsh, louder sounds with a moaning or snoring quality. Best heard on expiration but can be heard on both inspiration and expiration. May be altered by coughing	Air passing through narrowed air passages as a result of secretions, swelling, tumors	Loud sounds can be heard over most lung areas but predominate over the trachea and bronchi
Friction rub	Superficial grating or creaking sounds heard during inspiration and expiration. Not relieved by coughing	Rubbing together of inflamed pleural surfaces	Heard most often in areas of greatest thoracic expansion (e.g., lower anterior and lateral chest)
Wheeze	Continuous, high-pitched, squeaky musical sounds. Best heard on expiration. Not usually altered by coughing	Air passing through a constricted bronchus as a result of secretions, swelling, tumors	Heard over all lung fields; best heard on expiration

num and the clavicles. See Tables 2–1 and 2–2 for description of normal and adventitious breath sounds.

The Cardiovascular and Peripheral Vascular Systems

The Cardiovascular System

- Simultaneously inspect and palpate the precordium for the presence of abnormal pulsations, lifts, or heaves.
- Inspect and palpate the aortic, pulmonic, tricuspid, and apical areas for pulsations.
- Inspect and palpate the apical area for pulsation, noting its specific location and diameter.
- Auscultate the heart in all four anatomic sites: aortic, pulmonic, tricuspid, and apical (mitral). See Figure 2–2.
- Inspect and palpate the epigastric area (at the base of the sternum) for abdominal aortic pulsations.

The Peripheral Vascular System

- Palpate the peripheral pulses on both sides of the client's body systematically and simultaneously to determine the symmetry of pulse volume. If you have

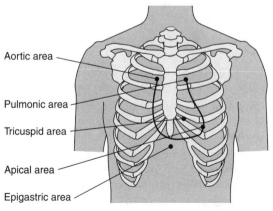

Aortic area

Pulmonic area

Tricuspid area

Apical area

Epigastric area

Figure 2–2 ■ Anatomic sites of the precordium.

difficulty palpating the peripheral pulses, use a Doppler ultrasound probe.

- Palpate the carotid arteries one at a time.
- Auscultate the carotid artery to determine the presence of a bruit.

Jugular Veins

- Inspect the jugular veins for distention while the client is in a semi-Fowler's position with the head supported on a small pillow.

Peripheral Veins

- Inspect the peripheral veins in the arms and legs for the presence or appearance of superficial veins when limbs are dependent and when limbs are elevated.
- Assess the peripheral leg veins for signs of phlebitis.

Peripheral Perfusion

- Inspect the skin of the hands and the feet for color, temperature, edema, and skin changes.
- Assess the adequacy of arterial flow if arterial insufficiency is suspected.

The Breasts and Axillae

- Use this as an opportunity to teach breast self-examination.
- Inspect and palpate the breasts of both men and women.
- Inspect the breasts for size, symmetry, and contour or shape while the client is in a sitting position.
- Inspect the skin of the breast for localized discolorations or hyperpigmentation, retraction or dimpling, localized hypervascular areas, swelling, or edema.
- Accentuate any retraction by having the client raise the arms above the head, push the hands together with elbows fixed, and/or press the hands down on the hips.
- Inspect the areola area for size, shape, symmetry, color, surface characteristics, and any masses or lesions.

- Palpate the axillary, subclavicular, and supraclavicular lymph nodes when the client is supine. Use the palmar surface of all fingertips to palpate.
- Palpate the breast for masses, tenderness, and any discharge from the nipples. Start at one point for palpation and move systematically to the end point to ensure that all breast surfaces are assessed.

The Abdomen
Inspection of the Abdomen
- Inspect the abdomen for skin integrity, contour, and symmetry.
- Observe abdominal movements associated with respiration, peristalsis, or aortic pulsations.

Auscultation of the Abdomen
- Auscultate the abdomen for bowel sounds, vascular sounds, and peritoneal friction rubs in all four quadrants. See Figure 2–3.

Palpation of the Abdomen
- Perform light palpation first to detect areas of tenderness and/or muscle guarding. Systematically explore all four quadrants.
- Perform deep palpation over all four quadrants.

Palpation of the Bladder
- Palpate the area above the pubic symphysis if the client's history indicates possible urinary retention.

The Musculoskeletal System
The Muscles
- Inspect muscles for size. Compare the muscles on one side of the body to the corresponding muscles on the other side.
- Inspect muscles and tendons for contractures.
- Inspect the muscles for fasciculations and tremors. Inspect any tremors by having the client hold the arms out in front of the body.
- Palpate the muscles at rest to determine muscle tonicity.

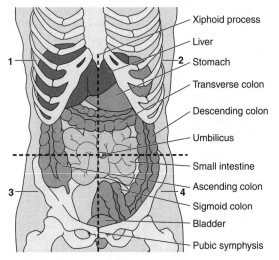

Figure 2–3 The four abdominal quadrants and the underlying organs. *1,* right upper quadrant; *2,* left upper quadrant; *3,* right lower quadrant; *4,* left lower quadrant.

- Palpate muscles while the client is active and passive for flaccidity, spasticity, and smoothness of movement.
- Test muscle strength. Compare the right side with the left side.

The Bones

- Inspect the skeleton for normal structure and deformities.
- Palpate the bones to locate any areas of edema or tenderness.

The Joints

- Inspect the joints for swelling.
- Palpate each joint for tenderness, smoothness of movement, swelling, crepitation, and the presence of nodules.
- Assess joint range of motion.

The Neurologic System
Gross Motor and Balance Test
Of the several gross motor function and balance tests, generally Romberg's test and one other are conducted. The following tests may be carried out.

- Romberg's test (Ask the client to stand with feet together and arms resting at the sides, first with eyes open, then closed. Stand close during this test to prevent the client from falling.)
- Walking gait
- Standing on one foot with eyes closed
- Heel–toe walking
- Toe or heel walking

Fine Motor Tests for the Upper Extremities
The following tests may be performed:

- Finger to nose
- Alternating supination and pronation of hands on knees
- Finger to nose and to the nurse's finger
- Finger to fingers
- Fingers to thumb (same hand)

Fine Motor Tests for the Lower Extremities
Ask the client to lie supine and perform these tests:

- Heel down opposite shin. Ask the client to place the heel of one foot just below the opposite knee and run the heel down the shin to the foot. Repeat with the other foot.
- Toe or ball of foot to the nurse's finger. Ask the client to touch your finger with the large toe of each foot.

Sensory Function

- Light-touch sensation. Compare the light-touch sensation of symmetric areas of the body.
- Pain sensation. Assess pain sensation by asking the client to close the eyes and report whether a sharp, dull, or indistinguishable sensation is felt when you

touch the skin with the sharp or dull end of an instrument. Alternate between the sharp and dull ends, and randomly select different anatomic sites. Do not perform this test on the face, however.

Temperature Sensation

- Temperature sensation is not routinely tested if the pain sensation is found to be within normal limits.
- If pain sensation is abnormal or absent, touch the skin areas with test tubes filled with warm or cold water. Have the client report whether a warm, cold, or indistinguishable sensation is felt.

Position or Kinesthetic Sensation

- Commonly, the middle fingers and the large toes are tested for the kinesthetic sensation (sense of position).
- Ask the client to close the eyes. Move the finger or toe until it is up, down, or straight out, and ask the client to identify the position.

Tactile Discrimination

For all tests, the client's eyes must be closed. The following tests may be performed:

- One- and two-point discrimination. Alternate touching the skin with one or two pins. Ask whether the client feels one or two pinpricks.
- Stereognosis. Place familiar objects (key, paper clip, or coin) in the client's hand, and ask the client to identify them. If the client has a motor impairment of the hand, write a number or letter on the hand with a blunt instrument, and ask the client to identify it.
- Extinction phenomenon. Simultaneously stimulate two symmetric areas of the body to determine whether both points of stimulus are felt.

The Female Genitals and Inguinal Lymph Nodes

- Inspect the distribution, amount, and characteristics of pubic hair.
- Inspect the skin of the pubic area for lesions, swelling, inflammation, and presence of parasites. To as-

sess adequately, separate the labia majora and labia minora.

- Inspect the clitoris, urethral orifice, and vaginal orifice when separating the labia minora.
- Palpate the inguinal lymph nodes using the pads of the fingers in a rotary motion, noting any enlargement or tenderness.

The Male Genitals and Inguinal Area

- Use this as an opportunity to teach testicular self-examination.
- Inspect pubic hair distribution, amount, and characteristics.
- Inspect the penile shaft and glans for lesions, nodules, swelling, and inflammation.
- Inspect the urethral meatus for swelling, inflammation, and discharge.
- Palpate the penis for tenderness, thickening, and nodules.
- Inspect the scrotum for appearance, size, and symmetry.
- Palpate the scrotum for masses, tenderness, or lesions.
- Palpate the scrotum to assess status of the underlying testes, epididymis, and spermatic cord.
- Inspect inguinal areas for bulges while the client is standing, if possible. Have the client hold the breath and strain or bear down as though having a bowel movement.
- Palpate hernias.

The Rectum and Anus

- Inspect the anus and surrounding tissue for color, integrity, and skin lesions.
- Palpate the rectum for anal sphincter tonicity, nodules, masses, and tenderness.
- On withdrawal of the gloved finger from the rectum and anus, observe it for feces.

Special Considerations for Assessment of Elders

History

- Allow extra time for clients to answer questions.
- Adapt questioning techniques as appropriate for clients with hearing or visual limitations.

The Skin

- Changes in white skin occur at an earlier age than in black skin.
- The skin loses its elasticity and wrinkles. Wrinkles first appear on the skin of the face and neck, which are abundant in collagen and elastic fibers.
- The skin appears thin and translucent because of loss of dermis and subcutaneous fat.
- The skin is dry and flaky because sebaceous and sweat glands are less active. Dry skin is more prominent over the extremities.
- The skin takes longer to return to its natural shape after being tented between the thumb and finger.
- Due to the normal loss of peripheral skin turgor in elders, assess for hydration by checking skin turgor over the sternum or clavicle.
- *Senile lentigines* or *melanotic freckles* are normally apparent on the back of the hand and other skin areas that are exposed to the sun.
- *Seborrheic keratosis* with irregularly shaped borders and a scaly surface often occurs on the face, shoulders, and trunk. These benign lesions begin as yellowish to tan and progress to a dark brown or black.
- *Vitiligo* tends to increase with age and is thought to result from an autoimmune response.
- Cutaneous tags are most commonly seen in the neck and axillary regions. These skin lesions vary in size and are soft, often flesh-colored, and pedicled.
- Visible, bright red, fine, dilated blood vessels (*telangiectasias*) commonly occur as a result of the thin-

ning of the dermis and the loss of support for the blood vessel walls.

- *Actinic keratoses* may appear at about age 50, often on the face, ears, backs of the hands, and arms. They may become malignant if untreated.

The Hair

- There may be loss of scalp, pubic, and axillary hair.
- In women, the hair of the eyebrows and some facial hair become coarse.
- In men, hairs of the eyebrows, ears, and nostrils become bristlelike and coarse.

The Nails

- The nails grow more slowly and thicken.
- Longitudinal bands commonly develop, and the nails tend to split.
- Bands across the nails may indicate protein deficiency; white spots, zinc deficiency; and spoon-shaped nails, iron deficiency.

The Eyes and Vision

- Visual acuity decreases as the lens of the eye ages and becomes more opaque and loses elasticity.
- The ability of the iris to accommodate to darkness and dim light diminishes.
- Peripheral vision diminishes.
- The adaptation to light (glare) and dark decreases.
- Accommodation to far objects often improves, but accommodation to near objects decreases.
- Color vision declines; older people are less able to perceive purple colors and to discriminate pastel colors.
- Many older people wear corrective lenses; they are most likely to have hyperopia. Visual changes are due to loss of elasticity (presbyopia) and transparency of the lens.
- The skin around the orbit of the eye may darken.
- The eyeball may appear sunken because of the decrease in orbital fat.

- Skinfolds of the upper lids may seem more prominent, and the lower lids may sag.

- The eyes may appear dry and lusterless because of the decrease in tear production from the lacrimal glands.

- *Arcus senilis* appears around part or all of the cornea. It results from an accumulation of a lipid substance on the cornea. The cornea tends to cloud with age.

- The iris may appear pale with brown discolorations as a result of pigment degeneration.

- The conjunctiva of the eye may appear paler than that of younger adults and may take on a slightly yellow appearance because of the deposition of fat.

- Pupil reaction to light and accommodation is normally symmetric but may be less brisk.

- The pupils can appear smaller in size, unequal, and irregular in shape because of sclerotic changes in the iris.

The Ears and Hearing

- The skin of the ear may appear dry and be less resilient because of the loss of connective tissue.

- Increased coarse and wirelike hair growth occurs along the helix, antihelix, and tragus.

- The pinna increases in both width and length, and the earlobe elongates.

- Earwax is drier.

- The tympanic membrane is more translucent and less flexible. The intensity of the light reflex may diminish slightly.

- Sensorineural hearing loss occurs.

- Generalized hearing loss (presbycusis) occurs in all frequencies, although the first symptom is the loss of high-frequency sounds: the *f, s, sh,* and *ph* sounds. To such persons, conversation can be distorted and result in what appears to be inappropriate or confused behavior.

The Mouth

- The oral mucosa may be drier than that of younger persons because of decreased salivary gland activity. Decreased salivation occurs only in elderly people taking prescribed medications such as antidepressants, antihistamines, decongestants, diuretics, antihypertensives, tranquilizers, antispasmodics, and antineoplastics. Extreme dryness is associated with dehydration.
- Some receding of the gums occurs, giving an appearance of increased toothiness.
- The gums may develop a brownish pigmentation, especially in blacks.
- Taste sensations diminish. Sweet and salty tastes are lost first. Elderly persons may add more salt and sugar to food than they did when they were younger. Diminished taste sensation is due to atrophy of the taste buds and a decreased sense of smell. It indicates diminished function of the fifth and seventh cranial nerves.
- Tiny purple or bluish-black swollen areas (varicosities) under the tongue, known as *caviar spots,* are not uncommon.
- The teeth may show signs of staining, erosion, chipping, and abrasions due to loss of dentin. Tooth loss occurs as a result of dental disease but is preventable with good dental hygiene.
- The gag reflex may be slightly sluggish.

The Thorax and Lungs

- The thoracic curvature may be accentuated (kyphosis) because of osteoporosis and changes in cartilage, resulting in collapse of the vertebrae.
- Kyphosis and osteoporosis alter the size of the chest cavity as the ribs move downward and forward.
- The anteroposterior diameter of the chest widens, giving a barrel-chested appearance.
- Breathing rate and rhythm are unchanged at rest; the rate normally increases with exercise but may take longer to return to the preexercise rate.

- Inspiratory muscles become less powerful, and the inspiration reserve volume decreases. A decrease in depth of respiration is therefore apparent.

- Expiration may require the use of accessory muscles. The expiratory reserve volume significantly increases because of the increased amount of air remaining in the lungs at the end of a normal breath.

- Deflation of the lung is incomplete.

- Small airways lose their cartilaginous support and elastic recoil; as a result, they tend to close, particularly in basal or dependent portions of the lung.

- Elastic tissue of the alveoli loses its stretchability and changes to fibrous tissue. Exertional capacity decreases.

- Cilia in the airways decrease in number and are less effective in removing mucus; elders are therefore at greater risk for pulmonary infections.

The Cardiovascular and Peripheral Vascular Systems

- Cardiac output and strength of contraction decrease, thus lessening the elder's activity tolerance.

- The heart rate returns to its resting rate more slowly after exertion than it did when the individual was younger.

- S_4 heart sound is considered normal in elders.

- Extra systoles commonly occur. Ten or more extra systoles per minute are considered abnormal.

- Sudden emotional and physical stresses may result in cardiac arrhythmias and heart failure.

- The overall effectiveness of blood vessels decreases as smooth muscle cells are replaced by connective tissue. The lower extremities are more likely to show signs of arterial and venous impairment because of the more distal and dependent position.

- Proximal arteries become thinner and dilate.

- Peripheral arteries become thicker and dilate less effectively because of arteriosclerotic changes in the vessel walls.

- Blood vessels lengthen and become more tortuous and prominent. Varicosities occur more frequently.

- In some instances, arteries may be palpated more easily because of the loss of supportive surrounding tissues. Often, however, the most distal pulses of the lower extremities are more difficult to palpate because of decreased arterial perfusion.

- Systolic and diastolic blood pressures increase, but the increase in the systolic pressure is greater. As a result, the pulse pressure widens. Any client with a blood pressure reading above 140/90 should be referred for follow-up assessments.

- Peripheral edema is frequently observed and is most commonly the result of chronic venous insufficiency or low protein levels in the blood (hypoproteinemia).

The Abdomen

- The rounded abdomens of elders are due to an increase in adipose tissue and a decrease in muscle tone.

- The abdominal wall is slacker and thinner, making palpation easier and more accurate than in younger clients. Muscle wasting and loss of fibroconnective tissue occur.

- The pain threshold in elders is often higher; major abdominal problems such as appendicitis or other acute emergencies may therefore go undetected.

- Gastrointestinal pain needs to be differentiated from cardiac pain. Gastrointestinal pain may be located in the chest or abdomen, whereas cardiac pain is usually located in the chest. Factors aggravating gastrointestinal pain are usually related to either ingestion or lack of food intake; gastrointestinal pain is usually relieved by antacids, food, or assuming an upright position. Common factors that can aggravate cardiac pain are activity or anxiety; rest or nitroglycerin relieves cardiac pain.

- Stool passes through the intestines at a slower rate in elders, and the perception of stimuli that produce the urge to defecate often diminishes.

- Fecal incontinence may occur in confused or neurologically impaired elders.

- The incidence of colon cancer is higher among elders than younger adults. Symptoms include a change in bowel function, rectal bleeding, and weight loss. Changes in bowel function, however, are associated with many factors, such as diet, exercise, and medications.

- Decreased absorption of oral medications often occurs with aging.

- In the liver, impaired metabolism of some drugs may occur with aging.

The Musculoskeletal System

- Muscle mass decreases progressively with age, although wide variations exist among different individuals.

- The decrease in speed, strength, resistance to fatigue, reaction time, and coordination in elders is due to a decrease in nerve conduction and muscle tone.

- The bones become more fragile, and osteoporosis leads to a loss of total bone mass. As a result, elders are predisposed to fractures and compressed vertebrae.

- In most elders, osteoarthritic changes in the joints can be observed.

The Neurologic System

- A full neurologic assessment can be lengthy. Conduct in several sessions if indicated and cease the tests if the client is noticeably fatigued.

- A decline in mental status is not a normal result of aging. Changes are more the result of physical or psychological disorders (e.g., fever, fluid and electrolyte imbalances).

- Intelligence and learning ability are unaltered with age. Many factors, however, inhibit learning (e.g., anxiety, illness, pain, cultural barrier).

- Short-term memory is often less efficient. Long-term memory is usually unaltered.

- Because old age is often associated with loss of support persons, depression is a common disorder. Mood changes, weight loss, anorexia, constipation, and early-morning awakening may manifest it.

- The stress of being in unfamiliar situations can cause confusion in elders.

- As a person ages, reflex responses may become less intense.

- Because elders tire more easily than younger clients, a total neurologic assessment is often done at a different time than the other parts of the physical assessment.

- Although there is a progressive decrease in the number of functioning neurons in the central nervous system and in the sense organs, the elder usually functions well because of the abundant reserves in the number of brain cells.

- Impulse transmission and reaction to stimuli are slower.

- Many elders have some impairment of hearing, vision, smell, temperature and pain sensation, memory, and mental endurance.

- Coordination changes, including a reduced speed of fine finger movements. Standing balance remains intact, and Romberg's test remains negative.

- Reflex responses may slightly increase or decrease. Many show loss of Achilles reflex, and the plantar reflex may be difficult to elicit.

- When testing sensory function, give elders time to respond. Normally, elders have unaltered perception of light touch and superficial pain, decreased perception of deep pain, and decreased perception of temperature stimuli. Many also reveal a decrease or absence of position sense in the large toes.

The Genitals

- Labia become atrophied and flatten.
- The clitoris is a common site for cancerous lesions.

- The vulva atrophies as a result of a reduction in vascularity, elasticity, adipose tissue, and estrogen levels. Because the vulva is more fragile, it is more easily irritated.

- The vaginal environment becomes drier and more alkaline, resulting in an alteration of the type of flora present and a predisposition to vaginitis. Dyspareunia (difficult or painful coitus) is also a common occurrence.

- The cervix and uterus decrease in size.

- The fallopian tubes and ovaries atrophy.

- Ovulation and estrogen production cease.

- Prolapse of the uterus occurs, especially in those who have had multiple pregnancies.

- The penis decreases in size with age; the size and firmness of the testes decrease.

- Testosterone is produced in smaller amounts.

- More time and direct physical stimulation are required for an elder to achieve an erection, but he can maintain the erection for a longer period before ejaculation than he could at a younger age.

- Seminal fluid is reduced in amount and viscosity.

- Urinary frequency, nocturia, dribbling, and problems with beginning and ending the stream are usually the result of prostatic enlargement.

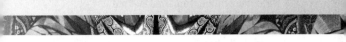

E. NURSING DIAGNOSES

North American Nursing Diagnosis Association (NANDA International) 2007–2008 Approved Nursing Diagnoses

Activity Intolerance

Activity Intolerance, Risk for

Airway Clearance, Ineffective

Anxiety

Anxiety, Death

Aspiration, Risk for

Attachment, Parent/Infant/Child, Risk for Impaired

Autonomic Dysreflexia

Autonomic Dysreflexia, Risk for

Blood Glucose, Risk for Unstable

Body Image, Disturbed

Body Temperature, Imbalanced, Risk for

Bowel Incontinence

Breast-feeding, Effective

Breast-feeding, Ineffective

Breast-feeding, Interrupted

Breathing Pattern, Ineffective

Cardiac Output, Decreased

Caregiver Role Strain

Caregiver Role Strain, Risk for

Comfort, Readiness for Enhanced

Communication, Impaired, Verbal

Communication, Readiness for Enhanced

Confusion, Acute

Confusion, Acute, Risk for

Confusion, Chronic

Constipation

Constipation, Perceived

Constipation, Risk for

Contamination

Contamination, Risk for

Coping, Community, Ineffective

Coping, Community, Readiness for Enhanced

Coping, Defensive

Coping, Family, Compromised

Coping, Family, Disabled

Coping, Family, Readiness for Enhanced

Coping, Individual, Readiness for Enhanced

Coping, Ineffective

Decisional Conflict

Decision Making, Readiness for Enhanced

Denial, Ineffective

Dentition, Impaired

Development, Delayed, Risk for

Diarrhea

Disuse Syndrome, Risk for

Diversional Activity, Deficient

Energy Field, Disturbed

Environmental Interpretation Syndrome, Impaired

Failure to Thrive, Adult

Falls, Risk for

Family Processes, Dysfunctional, Alcoholism

Family Processes, Interrupted

Family Processes, Readiness for Enhanced

Fatigue

Fear

Fluid Balance, Readiness for Enhanced

Fluid Volume, Deficient

Fluid Volume, Deficient, Risk for

Fluid Volume, Excess

Fluid Volume, Imbalanced, Risk for

Gas Exchange, Impaired

Grieving

Grieving, Complicated

Grieving, Risk for Complicated

Growth, Disproportionate, Risk for

Growth and Development, Delayed

Health Behavior, Risk-Prone

Health Maintenance, Ineffective

Health-Seeking Behaviors (Specify)

Home Maintenance, Impaired

Hope, Readiness for Enhanced

Hopelessness

Human Dignity, Risk for Compromised

Hyperthermia

Hypothermia

Immunization Status, Readiness for Enhanced

Infant Behavior, Disorganized

Infant Behavior, Disorganized, Risk for

Infant Behavior, Organized, Readiness for Enhanced

Infant Feeding Pattern, Ineffective

Infection, Risk for

Injury, Risk for

Insomnia

Intracranial Adaptive Capacity, Decreased

Knowledge, Deficient (Specify)

Knowledge, Readiness for Enhanced (Specify)

Latex Allergy Response

Latex Allergy Response, Risk for

Liver Function, Impaired, Risk for

Loneliness, Risk for

Memory, Impaired

Mobility, Bed, Impaired

Mobility, Physical, Impaired

Mobility, Wheelchair, Impaired

Moral Distress

Nausea

Neurovascular Dysfunction, Peripheral, Risk for

Noncompliance (Specify)

Nutrition, Imbalanced, Less than Body Requirements

Nutrition, Imbalanced, More than Body Requirements

Nutrition, Imbalanced, More than Body Requirements, Risk for

Nutrition, Readiness for Enhanced

Oral Mucous Membrane, Impaired

Pain, Acute

Pain, Chronic

Parenting, Impaired

Parenting, Readiness for Enhanced

Parenting, Risk for Impaired

Perioperative Positioning Injury, Risk for

Personal Identity, Disturbed

Poisoning, Risk for

Posttrauma Syndrome

Posttrauma Syndrome, Risk for

Power, Readiness for Enhanced

Powerlessness

Powerlessness, Risk for

Protection, Ineffective

Rape-Trauma Syndrome

Rape-Trauma Syndrome, Compound Reaction

Rape-Trauma Syndrome, Silent Reaction

Religiosity, Impaired

Religiosity, Readiness for Enhanced

Religiosity, Risk for Impaired

Relocation Stress Syndrome

Relocation Stress Syndrome, Risk for

Role Conflict, Parental

Role Performance, Ineffective

Sedentary Lifestyle

Self-Care, Readiness for Enhanced

Self-Care Deficit, Bathing/Hygiene

Self-Care Deficit, Dressing/Grooming

Self-Care Deficit, Feeding

Self-Care Deficit, Toileting

Self-Concept, Readiness for Enhanced

Self-Esteem, Chronic Low

Self-Esteem, Situational Low

Self-Esteem, Risk for Situational Low

Self-Mutilation

Self-Mutilation, Risk for

Sensory Perception, Disturbed (Specify: Auditory, Gustatory, Kinesthetic, Olfactory, Tactile, Visual)

Sexual Dysfunction

Sexuality Pattern, Ineffective

Skin Integrity, Impaired

Skin Integrity, Risk for Impaired

Sleep Deprivation

Sleep, Readiness for Enhanced

Social Interaction, Impaired

Social Isolation

Sorrow, Chronic

Spiritual Distress

Spiritual Distress, Risk for

Spiritual Well-Being, Readiness for Enhanced

Spontaneous Ventilation, Impaired

Stress, Overload

Sudden Infant Death Syndrome, Risk for

Suffocation, Risk for

Suicide, Risk for

Surgical Recovery, Delayed

Swallowing, Impaired

Therapeutic Regimen Management, Community, Ineffective

Therapeutic Regimen Management, Effective

Therapeutic Regimen Management, Family, Ineffective

Therapeutic Regimen Management, Ineffective

Therapeutic Regimen Management, Readiness for Enhanced

Thermoregulation, Ineffective

Thought Processes, Disturbed

Tissue Integrity, Impaired

Tissue Perfusion, Ineffective (Specify: Cerebral, Cardiopulmonary, Gastrointestinal, Renal)

Tissue Perfusion, Ineffective, Peripheral

Transfer Ability, Impaired

Trauma, Risk for

Unilateral Neglect

Urinary Elimination, Impaired

Urinary Elimination, Readiness for Enhanced

Urinary Incontinence, Functional

Urinary Incontinence, Overflow

Urinary Incontinence, Reflex

Urinary Incontinence, Stress

Urinary Incontinence, Total

Urinary Incontinence, Urge

Urinary Incontinence, Risk for Urge

Urinary Retention

Ventilatory Weaning Response, Dysfunctional

Violence, Other-Directed, Risk for

Violence, Self-Directed, Risk for

Walking, Impaired

Wandering

Note: From *NANDA Nursing Diagnoses: Definitions and Classification, 2007–2008.* Philadelphia: North American Nursing Diagnosis Association. Used with permission.

Formulating Diagnostic Statements

The basic two-part statement includes the following:

1. *Problem (P):* statement of the client's response (NANDA label)

2. *Etiology (E):* factors contributing to or probable causes of the responses

Sample Two-Part Diagnostic Statements

Problem	Related to	Etiology
Constipation	Related to	Prolonged laxative use
Severe anxiety	Related to	Threat to physiologic integrity: possible cancer diagnosis

The basic three-part nursing diagnosis statement is called the *PES format* and includes the following:

1. *Problem (P):* statement of the client's response (NANDA label)

2. *Etiology (E):* factors contributing to or probable causes of the response

3. *Signs and symptoms (S):* defining characteristics manifested by the client

Sample Three-Part Diagnostic Statement

Problem	Related to	Etiology	As Manifested by	Signs and Symptoms
Situational low self-esteem	Related to (r/t)	Feelings of rejection by husband	As manifested by (a.m.b.)	Hypersensitivity to criticism; states "I don't know if I can manage by myself" and rejects positive feedback

PLANNING AND IMPLEMENTATION

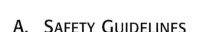

A. SAFETY GUIDELINES

To be a safe practitioner, you must know your limitations, know how and when to seek information, and stay current in your field. As health care advances, techniques are modified. Attend the classes, read the literature, and become familiar with your responsibilities as set forth by your agency. For example, cardiopulmonary resuscitation certification is required by most health care facilities; do not allow your certification to lapse.

Many health care agencies also have specific guidelines or procedures to follow in the event of an emergency, such as fire. Familiarize yourself with this information each time you go to a new facility. On each unit, make sure you know the location of the exit doors, the stairs, the crash cart, and the fire extinguishers. The first rule of safety is preparedness.

Know your resources. Find out where on the unit the procedure manuals are kept. If you are unfamiliar with a procedure, look it up. Knowing your resources also means knowing to whom you can go with questions or whom to seek out for advice. Your clinical instructor is one of your best safety resources. This person knows your level of knowledge, your clinical skill level, and your anxiety level. If you have concerns, talk them out with your instructor. Never perform skills that you are unsure of; always review the skill and seek assistance if you feel uncertain. See Chapter 32 of *Fundamentals of Nursing* for a thorough discussion of safety guidelines.

Investigate the availability of resource manuals. Does your unit have a *Physicians' Desk Reference* or drug handbook? Be familiar with all medications that you administer: Carry a drug handbook, or consult a unit handbook before administering medications. If you still have questions, go to your instructor for help. Be aware that the pharmacy staff is there to help you; pharmacists are particularly helpful for answering questions about new drugs, discussing drug–drug interactions, and planning medication schedules for clients.

Do not take unnecessary risks. Follow standard precautions to protect yourself from bloodborne pathogens. See pages 140 to 147 for a quick reference on standard precautions. To provide safe care, you must also use good body mechanics. Even when using good body mechanics, the average nurse should not lift more than 51 pounds and only under very controlled circumstances. The development of assistive client handling equipment and devices has rendered strict "manual" client handling unnecessary. Summaries of body mechanics guidelines and other safety guidelines are provided next.

Guidelines Related to Body Mechanics

- Start any body movement with proper alignment.

- Stand as close as possible to the object to be moved.

- Avoid stretching, reaching, and twisting, which may place the line of gravity outside your base of support.

- Before moving objects, increase your stability by widening your stance and flexing your knees, hips, and ankles.

- Adjust the working area to waist level, and keep your body close to the area.

- To prevent stretching and reaching, elevate adjustable beds and overbed tables, or lower the side rails of beds.

- When pushing an object, enlarge your base of support by moving your front foot forward.

- When pulling an object, enlarge your base of support either by moving the rear leg back (if you are facing the object) or by moving the front foot forward (if you are facing away from the object).

- Before moving objects, contract your gluteal, abdominal, leg, and arm muscles to prepare them for action.
- To move objects below your center of gravity, begin with the back and knees flexed. When lifting the weight, use your gluteal and leg muscles rather than the sacrospinal muscles of your back to exert an upward thrust.
- To prevent back strain, distribute the workload between both arms and legs.
- Always face the direction of the movement to prevent twisting of the spine and ineffective use of major muscle groups.
- When moving or carrying objects, hold them as close as possible to your center of gravity.
- To control an object's movement and keep it close to your center of gravity, pull the object toward you when possible rather than pushing it away.
- Provide a firm, smooth, dry foundation before moving a client in bed.
- Pull clients rather than push them when possible.
- Encourage clients to assist as much as possible by pushing or pulling themselves to reduce the muscular effort you need to expend.
- Use arms as levers when possible to increase lifting power.
- Use your own body weight to counteract the weight of the object you are moving. For example, lean forward when pushing an object, and rock your body weight backward when pulling an object or client toward you.
- Obtain the assistance of other persons or use mechanical devices to move objects that are too heavy for you to move alone.
- Avoid working against gravity.

- Pull, push, roll, or turn objects instead of lifting them.
- Lower the head of the client's bed before moving the client up in bed.
- Alternate rest periods with periods of muscle use to help prevent fatigue.

Preventing Falls in Hospitals

- Orient clients upon admission to their surroundings, and explain the call system.
- Carefully assess the client's ability to ambulate and transfer; provide walking aids and assistance as required.
- Closely supervise the clients at risk for falls during the first few days, especially at night.
- Encourage the client to use the call bell to request assistance; ensure that the bell is within reach.
- Place bedside tables and overbed tables near the bed or chair so that clients do not overreach and consequently lose their balance.
- Always keep hospital beds in the low position when not providing care so that clients can move into or out of bed easily.
- Encourage clients to use grab bars mounted in toilet and bathing areas and railings along corridors.
- Make sure nonskid bath mats are available in tubs and showers.
- Encourage the client to wear nonskid footwear.
- Keep the environment tidy, especially keep light cords from underfoot and furniture out of the way.
- Reduce poor lighting and glare, which causes clients to squint.
- Use individualized interventions (e.g., alarm sensitive to client position) rather than side rails for confused clients.

Adult Home Hazard Appraisal

- *Walkways and stairways (inside and outside).* Note uneven sidewalks or paths, broken or loose steps, absence of handrails or placement on only one side of stairways, insecure handrails, congested hallways or other traffic areas, and adequacy of lighting at night.

- *Floors.* Note uneven and highly polished or slippery floors and any unanchored rugs or mats.

- *Furniture.* Note hazardous placement of furniture with sharp corners. Note chairs or stools that are too low to get into and out of or that provide inadequate support.

- *Bathroom(s).* Note the presence of grab bars around tubs and toilets, nonslip surfaces in tubs and shower stalls, adequacy of lighting for medicine cabinet, and need for raised toilet seat or bath chair in tub or shower.

- *Kitchen.* Note pilot lights (gas stove) in need of repair, inaccessible storage areas, and hazardous furniture. Check for presence of operational smoke detector.

- *Bedrooms.* Note adequacy of lighting, in particular the availability of night-lights and accessibility of light switches. Assess floors and furniture as previously. Note access to bathroom.

- *Electrical.* Note unanchored and/or frayed electrical cords, overloaded outlets, and any outlets near water.

- *Fire protection.* Note the presence or absence of a fire extinguisher and fire escape plan, improper storage of combustibles (e.g., gasoline) or corrosives [e.g., rust remover (phosphoric acid)], and accessibility of emergency telephone numbers (fire, police).

- *Toxic substances.* Note appropriate storage of medicines or toxic substances such as cleaning solutions. Note medications kept beyond date of expiration and improperly labeled cleaning solutions.

Steps to Follow in the Event of Fire

- Activate the fire alarm if one is nearby.
- Notify the hospital switchboard of the location of the fire.

- Evacuate clients who are in immediate danger. First, direct ambulatory clients to a safe area, or enlist their help in moving clients in wheelchairs. This clears the area for the evacuation of nonambulatory clients, who can be moved in a stretcher or bed, carried, or dragged on sheets and blankets.
- If the fire is small, use the fire extinguisher.
- Close windows and doors in the area of the fire to reduce ventilation.
- Turn off oxygen and any electrical appliances in the vicinity.
- Clear fire exits, if necessary.
- Contain smoke as necessary by placing damp cloths or blankets around the outside edges of doors.
- Protect clients from smoke inhalation by giving them wet washcloths through which to breathe.

Discharge Planning and Home Care Assessment

Client/Environment
- Self-care abilities for hygiene and toileting
- Self-care abilities for medication administration
- Self-care abilities for wound care
- Facilities: presence of running water, garbage, bathroom to facilitate wound care and contain potentially infectious materials

Family
- Caregiver availability, skills, and willingness
- Family concerns about caregiving

Community
- Resources

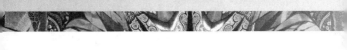

B. CLINICAL GUIDELINES

1. Fluid and Electrolyte Balance
Assess to Determine

- The usual amount and type of fluids ingested each day
- Foods rich in protein, sodium, potassium, and calcium eaten each day
- Any recent changes in food or fluid intake and reason (e.g., presence of nausea, pain, anorexia, or dysphagia)
- Any recent changes in frequency or amount of urine output
- Major losses of body fluid through vomiting, diarrhea, excessive perspiration, or other route (e.g., drainage from gastrointestinal function, ileostomy, colostomy, or burn sites)
- History of any long-term or recent disease processes that might disrupt fluid, electrolyte, and acid–base balance: kidney disease, heart disease, high blood pressure, diabetes mellitus, diabetes insipidus, thyroid or parathyroid disorders, asthma, emphysema, severe trauma, or other chronic disease states (e.g., cancer, colitis, ileitis)
- Medication therapy that could affect fluid and electrolyte balance: diuretics, steroids, potassium supplements, or aldosterone inhibitor agents
- Recent treatments that could affect fluid and electrolyte balance, such as dialysis, total parenteral nutrition, tube drainage (e.g., nasogastric or intestinal suction), or tube feedings

Assess the Client for

- Signs that indicate insufficient hydration: excessive thirst, dry skin and mucous membranes, concentrated urine, reduced urine output, poor tissue turgor, depressed periorbital spaces
- Signs indicating excessive hydration: swollen ankles, difficulty breathing, sudden weight gain, ascites, moist crackles (rales) in lungs
- Signs that might indicate an electrolyte or acid–base imbalance: loss of mental alertness; disorientation; faintness; muscle weakness, twitching, cramps, fatigue, pain, or spasm; abnormal sensations (e.g., burning, prickling, tingling); abdominal cramps or distention; heart palpitations

Obtain Clinical Measurements

- *Baseline and daily weight.* Rapid losses or gains of 5% or more of total body weight indicate moderate to severe fluid volume deficit or excess.
- *Vital signs. Body temperature*: An increased body temperature may indicate hypernatremic dehydration; a decreased body temperature may result from hypovolemia. *Pulse rate*: An increased pulse rate and a weak, thready pulse may occur with fluid volume deficit or potassium excess. *Respiration*: An increased rate and depth of respiration may cause carbonic acid deficit (respiratory alkalosis); shallow respirations may create a carbonic acid excess (respiratory acidosis). Either may be a compensatory mechanism for metabolic acid–base imbalances. *Blood pressure*: An elevated systolic blood pressure may indicate a fluid volume excess; a sudden decreased systolic pressure exceeding 10 mm Hg usually indicates a fluid volume deficit.
- Twenty-four–hour fluid intake and output.

Review Results of Laboratory Tests

- Serum electrolyte levels
- Hematocrit
- Urine pH

- Urine specific gravity
- Arterial blood gases

Identify Clients at Risk for Fluid and Electrolyte Imbalances

- Postoperative clients
- Clients with severe trauma or burns
- Clients with chronic diseases, such as heart failure, diabetes, chronic obstructive lung disease, and cancer
- Clients who are permitted nothing by mouth
- Clients with intravenous infusions
- Clients with retention catheters and urinary drainage systems
- Clients with special drainages or suctions, such as a nasogastric suction
- Clients receiving diuretics
- Clients experiencing excessive fluid losses and requiring increased intake
- Clients who retain fluids
- Clients with fluid restrictions
- Elders who may not be taking in the fluids they need
- Clients unable to respond to the thirst sensation (e.g., comatose clients)
- Clients receiving electrolyte therapy (e.g., potassium supplements)
- Clients unable to communicate desire for fluid (e.g., very young and elderly clients)
- Clients with very high or very low total body water

Monitoring Fluid Intake and Output

- To assess fluid balance, determine the client's intake and output, and observe the client for signs of dehydration or overhydration.
- Monitor intake and output for all clients (a) whose oral fluid intake is insufficient, (b) who are experiencing excessive fluid loss via normal or abnormal

routes, (c) who are retaining fluid, or (d) who are taking medications that alter fluid output.

- Weigh clients who are retaining fluid or receiving diuretics daily.

Facilitating Normal or Increased Fluid Intake

- Explain to the client the reason for the required intake and the specific amount needed. This gives the client a rationale for the requirement and thus promotes compliance.

- Establish a 24-hour plan for ingesting the fluids. Generally, half of the total volume is ingested during the day shift, and the other half is divided between the evening and night shifts, with the majority ingested during the evening shift. For example, if 2500 mL is to be ingested in 24 hours, the plan may specify that 1500 mL be ingested in the 7-to-3 shift, 700 mL in the 3-to-11 shift, and 300 mL in the 11-to-7 shift. To prevent the need to urinate during sleeping hours, clients should avoid ingesting large amounts of fluid before bedtime.

- Set short-term outcomes that the client can realistically meet. For example, the client might ingest a glass of fluid every hour while awake or a pitcher of water by noon.

- Identify fluids the client likes, and make available a variety of those items. Examples may include fruit juices, tea, coffee, and milk (if allowed).

- Help clients to select foods that tend to become liquid at room temperature (e.g., gelatin, ice cream, sherbert, custard), if these are allowed.

- For clients who are confined to bed, supply appropriate cups, glasses, and straws to facilitate appropriate fluid intake. Keep the fluids within easy reach.

- Make sure fluids are served at the appropriate temperature: hot fluids hot, and cold fluids iced and cold.

- Encourage clients to participate in maintaining the fluid intake record, when possible. This helps them determine whether they are achieving preestablished goals.

- Be alert for the cultural implications of food and fluids. Some cultures may restrict certain foods and fluids and view others as having healing properties.

Helping Clients Restrict Fluid Intake

- Explain the reason for the restricted intake and how much and what types of fluids are permitted orally. Many clients need to be informed that ice chips, gelatin, and ice cream, for example, are considered fluid.

- Help the client decide how to allocate the total amount of fluid allowed: how much to take with each meal, between meals, before bedtime, and with medications. Generally, half of the total volume is scheduled during the day shift, when the client is most active, receives two meals, and, often, most oral medications. A large part of the remainder is scheduled for the evening shift to permit the client to take fluids with meals and during evening visits.

- Identify fluids the client likes, and make sure that these are provided, unless contraindicated. A client who is allowed only 200 mL of fluid for breakfast, for example, should receive the type of fluid the client favors.

- Set short-term goals that make the fluid restriction more tolerable. For example, schedule a specified amount of fluid at 1- or 2-hour intervals between meals. Some clients may prefer fluids between meals only, because the food provided at mealtime may help relieve feelings of thirst.

- Provide the client with small fluid containers that make the container appear to contain more fluid than it actually does.

- Periodically offer the client ice chips as an alternative to water. Ice chips occupy twice the volume of an equal amount of water.

- Help clients rinse their mouths with water if they can do so without swallowing the fluid.

- Ensure meticulous oral care.
- Instruct the client to avoid ingesting or chewing salty or sweet foods (hard candy or gum) because these foods tend to produce thirst. Sugarless gum may be an alternative for some clients.
- Encourage the client to participate in maintaining the fluid intake record, when possible.

Special Care for Elders
Fluid and Electrolyte Balance

Certain changes related to aging place the elder at risk for serious problems with fluid and electrolyte imbalance, if homeostatic mechanisms are compromised. These changes include decreases in the following:

- Thirst sensation
- Ability of the kidneys to concentrate urine
- Intracellular fluid and total body water
- Response to body hormones that help regulate fluid and electrolytes

Other factors that may influence fluid and electrolyte balance in elders are the following:

- Increased use of diuretics for hypertension and heart disease
- Decrease in fluid and food intake, especially in elders with dementia or who are dependent on others to feed them and offer them fluids
- Preparations for certain diagnostic tests that have the client take nothing by mouth for long periods of time or cause diarrhea from laxative preparations
- Clients with impaired renal function, such as elderly clients and/or those with diabetes
- Those having certain diagnostic procedures. (Dyes used for some procedures, such as arteriograms and cardiac catheterizations, may cause further renal problems. Always see that the client is well hydrated before, during, and after the procedure to help in diluting and excreting the dye. If the client can take nothing by mouth for the

procedure, the nurse should check with the primary care provider to see if intravenous fluids are needed.)

- Any condition that may tax the normal compensatory mechanisms, such as a fever, influenza, surgery, or heat exposure

These conditions increase the elder's risk for fluid and electrolyte imbalance. The change can happen quickly and become serious in a short time. Astute observations and quick actions by the nurse can help prevent serious consequences. A change in mental status may be the first symptom of impairment and must be further evaluated to determine the cause.

2. Individualizing Care for Clients with Pain

- Establish a trusting relationship. Convey your concern and acknowledge that you believe the client is experiencing pain. A trusting relationship encourages the client to express thoughts and feelings and enhances the effectiveness of planned pain therapies.

- Assess the source of the pain carefully. The source of the pain may not always be what is apparent. For example, the postoperative client who has had abdominal surgery may complain of pain related to a headache or other discomfort.

- Consider the client's ability and willingness to participate actively in pain-relief measures. Excessively fatigued or sedated clients or those who have altered levels of consciousness are less able to actively participate.

- Use a variety of pain relief measures. It is thought that using more than one measure has an additive effect in relieving pain. Two measures that should always be part of a pain relief plan are (a) establishing a trusting client–nurse relationship and (b) client teaching. Because a client's pain may vary throughout a 24-hour period, different types of pain relief are often indicated during that time.

- Provide measures to relieve pain before it becomes severe. For example, it is better to provide an analgesic before pain is expected than to wait for the client to complain of pain, when a larger dose may be required.

- Use pain relief measures that the client believes are effective. It has been recognized that clients are often knowledgeable about measures that are effective in relieving their own pain. Therefore, incorporate the client's measures into a pain relief plan, unless they are harmful.

- Consider the client's willingness to participate actively in pain-relief measures.

- Base the choice of the pain-relief measure on the client's report of the severity of the pain. If a client reports mild pain, an analgesic such as aspirin may be indicated, whereas a client who reports severe pain may require a more potent relief measure.

- If a pain-relief measure proves to be ineffective, encourage the client to try it once or twice more before abandoning it. Anxiety may inhibit the effectiveness of a pain-relief measure, and some approaches, such as distraction strategies, require practice before they become effective.

- Maintain an unbiased attitude (open mind) about what may relieve the pain. New ways to relieve pain are continually being developed. It is not always possible to explain why a pain-relief measure works; however, you should support a measure unless it is harmful.

- Keep trying. Do *not* ignore a client because pain persists in spite of taking measures to relieve it. In these circumstances, reassess the pain, and consider other pain-relief measures.

- Prevent harm to the client. Pain therapy should not increase discomfort or harm the client.

- Educate the client and support persons about pain. Inform them about possible causes, precipitating and alleviating factors, and alternatives to drug therapy. Correct any misconceptions.

Pain-Distraction Techniques

- *Slow, rhythmic breathing.* Instruct the client to stare at an object, inhale slowly through the nose while counting from 1 to 4, and then exhale slowly through the mouth while counting to 4 again. Encourage the client to concentrate on the sensation of breathing and to picture a restful scene. Continue until a rhythmic pattern is established.

- *Massage and slow, rhythmic breathing.* Instruct the client to breathe rhythmically while massaging a painful body part with stroking or circular movements.

- *Rhythmic singing and tapping.* Ask the client to select a well-liked song and focus attention on its words and rhythm. Encourage the client to mouth or sing the words and tap a finger or foot. Loud, fast songs are best for intense pain.

- *Active listening.* Have the client listen to music and concentrate on the rhythm by tapping a finger or foot.

- *Guided imagery.* Ask the client to close the eyes and imagine and describe something pleasurable. As the client describes the image, ask about the sights, sounds, and smells imagined, encouraging the client to provide details.

Special Care for Elders
Pain Management

- Focus on the client's control in dealing with the pain.
- Spend time with the client and listen carefully.
- Clarify misconceptions. Encourage independence when possible.

Patient-Controlled Analgesia Pump

- Carefully monitor for drug side effects.
- Use cautiously for individuals with impaired pulmonary or renal function.
- Assess the client's cognitive and physical ability to use the client control button.

3. Respiratory Function

Assess to Determine

- *Current respiratory problems.* What recent changes has the client experienced in breathing pattern (e.g., shortness of breath, difficulty breathing, need to be in upright position to breathe, or rapid and shallow breathing)?

- *History of respiratory disease.* Has the client had colds, allergies, croup, asthma, tuberculosis, bronchitis, pneumonia, or emphysema? How frequently have these occurred? How long did they last? How were they treated?

- *Presence of a cough.* Is the cough productive or nonproductive? If productive, when is sputum produced? What are the amount, color, thickness, odor, and character of the sputum (e.g., thick, frothy, pink, rusty, or blood-tinged)?

- *Lifestyle.* Does the client smoke? If so, what (cigarettes, pipe, cigar) and how much? Does any member of the client's family smoke? Are there any occupational hazards (e.g., noxious fumes)?

- *Pain.* Does the client experience any pain associated with breathing or activity? Where is the pain located? What words does the client use to describe the pain? How long does it last, and how does it affect breathing? What activities precede the pain?

- *Medication history.* Has the client taken or does the client take any over-the-counter or prescription medications for breathing? Which ones? What are the dosages, times taken, and effects on the client, including side effects?

Observe the Client's

- Breathing pattern (rate, rhythm, depth, and quality). Note any signs of hyperventilation or hypoventilation, tachypnea, or bradypnea.

- Ease or effort of breathing and posture assumed for breathing (e.g., orthopneic).

- Breath sounds audible without amplification (e.g., stridor, stertor, wheeze, bubbling).
- Chest movements (e.g., retractions, flail chest, or paradoxical breathing). Note the specific location of retractions: intercostal, substernal, suprasternal, or supraclavicular.
- Clinical signs of hypoxia or anoxia, such as increased pulse rate, rapid or deep respirations, cyanosis of the skin and nail beds, restlessness, anxiety, dizziness (vertigo), or faintness (syncope).
- The location of any surgical incision in relation to the muscles needed for breathing. An incision can impede appropriate lung expansion.

Palpate the Chest for
- Respiratory excursion
- Vocal (tactile) fremitus

Percuss the Chest for
- Diaphragmatic excursion
- Chest sounds (flatness, dullness, resonance, hyperresonance, tympany)

Auscultate the Lungs for
- Breath sounds (normal, adventitious, or absent). See the tables on pages 39 and 40.

Determine the Results of
- Sputum analysis
- Venous blood samples (e.g., complete blood count)
- Arterial blood samples (blood gases)
- Pulmonary function tests
- Pulse oximetry

Abnormal Breathing Patterns and Breath Sounds
Breathing Patterns

Rate
- Tachypnea—quick, shallow breaths
- Bradypnea—abnormally slow breathing
- Apnea—cessation of breathing

Volume

- Hyperventilation—overexpansion of the lungs characterized by rapid and deep breaths
- Hypoventilation—underexpansion of the lungs, characterized by shallow respirations

Rhythm

- Cheyne-Stokes breathing—rhythmic waxing and waning of respirations, from very deep to very shallow breathing and temporary apnea

Ease or Effort

- Dyspnea—difficult and labored breathing during which the individual has a persistent, unsatisfied need for air and feels distressed
- Orthopnea—ability to breathe only in upright sitting or standing positions

Breath Sounds

Audible without Amplification

- Stridor—a shrill, harsh sound heard during inspiration with laryngeal obstruction
- Stertor—snoring or sonorous respiration, usually due to a partial obstruction of the upper airway
- Wheeze—continuous, high-pitched musical squeak or whistling sound occurring on expiration and sometimes on inspiration when air moves through a narrowed or partially obstructed airway
- Bubbling—gurgling sounds heard as air passes through moist secretions in the respiratory tract

Audible by Stethoscope

- Crackles (rales)—dry or wet crackling sounds similar to the sound produced by rolling a lock of hair near the ear; generally heard on inspiration as air moves through accumulated moist secretions
- Gurgles (rhonchi)—coarse, leathery, or grating sound produced by the rubbing together of inflamed pleural tissues

Chest Movements

- Intercostal retraction—indrawing between the ribs

- Substernal retraction—indrawing beneath the breastbone
- Suprasternal retraction—indrawing above the clavicles

Secretions and Coughing

- Hemoptysis—the presence of blood in the sputum
- Productive cough—a cough accompanied by expectorated secretions
- Nonproductive cough—a dry, harsh cough without secretions

Oropharyngeal and Nasopharyngeal Suctioning

- Assess for clinical signs indicating the need for suctioning: restlessness; gurgling sounds during respiration; adventitious breath sounds when the chest is auscultated; change in mental status, skin color, rate and pattern of respirations, pulse rate, and rhythm. Reassess these after suctioning.
- Hyperventilate and hyperoxygenate the client before and after suctioning.
- In the unconscious client, prevent aspiration of sputum by positioning the person in the lateral position.
- Maintain sterility of the suction catheter, flushing solution, and gauzes used to wipe the catheter.
- Before the procedure, measure the correct length for catheter insertion.
- Moisten the catheter tip before insertion.
- Insert the catheter without applying suction. For tracheal suctioning, insert the catheter while the client inhales.
- Never force the catheter against an obstruction.
- Gently rotate the catheter while applying suction.
- Prevent or minimize hypoxia: Apply suction for no more than 15 seconds each time. Allow 20- to 30-second intervals between each suction, and limit suctioning to 5 minutes in total.
- Encourage deep breathing and coughing between suctions.

- Flush the catheter between suctions.
- Change suction collection bottles and tubing at least daily.

Special Care for Elders

- Elders often have cardiac and/or pulmonary disease, thus increasing their susceptibility to hypoxemia related to suctioning. Watch closely for signs of hypoxemia. If noted, stop suctioning and hyperoxygenate.

4. Tube Feedings

Assess to Determine

- *Allergies to any food in the feeding.* Common ingredients in feedings include milk, sugar, water, eggs, and vegetable oil.
- *Bowel sounds before each feeding* (or every 4 to 8 hours for continuous feedings) to determine intestinal activity.
- *Abdominal distention at least daily.* Measure the client's abdominal girth at the umbilicus. A distended abdomen may indicate intolerance to a previous feeding.
- *Presence of regurgitation and feelings of fullness after feedings.*
- *Dumping syndrome.* Jejunostomy clients may experience nausea, vomiting, diarrhea, cramps, pallor, sweating, heart palpitations, increased pulse rate, and fainting after a feeding. Dumping syndrome results when hypertonic foods and liquids suddenly distend the jejunum. Smaller, more frequent feedings, and slower feedings may relieve dumping.
- *Presence of diarrhea, constipation, or flatulence.* The lack of bulk in liquid feedings may cause constipation. The presence of concentrated ingredients may cause diarrhea and flatulence.
- *Hydration status.* Measure the client's fluid intake and output, and note complaints of thirst. Additional water may need to be instilled between feedings.

Inserting a Nasogastric Tube

- Minimize discomfort by positioning the client appropriately, lubricating the tube, and working cooperatively with the client.
- Never force the tube against resistance.
- Confirm correct placement of the tube according to agency policy. Aspirate stomach contents, and check the pH, which should be acidic. X-ray and carbon dioxide detection may also be used.
- Secure the tube appropriately to the client's nose or nose and cheek.

Administering a Nasogastric or Orogastric Feeding
Before Administering the Feeding

- Assess the client for feelings of abdominal distention, belching, loose stools, flatus, or pain; assess the client for bowel sounds and allergies to foods in the feeding.
- Check the expiration date of the feeding.
- Warm the feeding to room temperature.
- Position the client in Fowler's or right lateral position.
- Confirm correct placement of the tube.

    1. Aspirate 20 to 30 mL of gastrointestinal secretions. Gastric secretions tend to be a grassy-green, off-white, or tan color; intestinal fluid is stained with bile and has a golden yellow or brownish-green color.

    2. Measure the pH of aspirated fluid.

        - Gastric aspirates have a pH of 1 to 4 but may be as high as 6 if the client is receiving medications that control gastric acid.
        - Small intestine aspirates generally have a pH of 6 or higher.
        - Respiratory secretions have a pH of 7 or higher. There is a possibility of respiratory placement when the pH reading is as low as 6.

- Therefore, when pH readings are 6 or higher, radiographic confirmation of tube location needs to be considered, especially in clients with diminished cough and gag reflexes.

3. Auscultate the epigastrium while injecting 5 to 20 mL of air. Air injected into the stomach produces whooshing, gurgling, or bubbling sounds over the epigastrium and the upper left quadrant. Accuracy of this method in predicting placement is less reliable than pH testing.

- Aspirate all residual stomach contents; measure the amount. Check agency policy to determine whether to reinstill the contents or to continue the feeding.
- Remove air from the tubing.
- Deliver the feeding over the desired length of time.

During the Feeding

- If the client is on a continuous feeding, check the gastric residual every 4 to 6 hours or according to agency protocol.

After the Feeding

- Flush the nasogastric tube with water.
- Clamp the nasogastric tube before all of the rinse solution has run through.
- Have the client remain in Fowler's position or a slightly elevated right lateral position for at least 30 minutes.

Removing a Nasogastric Tube

- If present, turn off the suction, and disconnect the tube from suction.
- Clamp the tubing.
- Remove the adhesive tape securing the tube to the nose.
- Don disposable gloves.
- Ask the client to take a deep breath and to hold it. Quickly and smoothly, withdraw the tube.

Administering a Gastrostomy or Jejunostomy Feeding

Before the Feeding

- Position the client appropriately.
- Assess the peristomal skin.
- Lubricate tubes before inserting them into stomas.
- Aspirate, measure, and reinstill (if indicated) stomach or jejunal contents. Check agency policy to confirm whether the feeding is to be withheld if more than 50 mL of stomach or jejunal contents is aspirated.

After the Feeding

- Rinse the tube with water.
- Have the client remain in Fowler's position or a slightly elevated right lateral position for at least 30 minutes.
- Clean the peristomal skin, and inspect for irritation.
- Apply peristomal skin protectants and appropriate dressings.

Special Care for Elders

- Physiologic changes associated with aging may make the elder more vulnerable to complications associated with enteral feedings. Decreased gastric emptying may necessitate checking frequently for gastric residual. Diarrhea from administering the feeding too fast or too high concentration of the feeding may cause dehydration in the elder. If the feeding has a high concentration of glucose, assess for hyperglycemia, as with aging there is decreased ability to handle increased glucose levels.

- Conditions such as hiatal hernia and diabetes mellitus may cause the stomach to empty more slowly. This increases the risk of aspiration in a client receiving a tube feeding. Checking for gastric residual more frequently can help document this if it is an ongoing problem. Changing the formula, altering the rate of administration, repositioning the client, or obtaining a physician's order for a medication to increase stomach emptying may resolve this problem.

5. Urinary Elimination

Assess to Determine

- Client's usual patterns and frequency of urination. Ask at what approximate times voiding occurs each day.

Note Recent Alterations in Voiding

- Passage of unusually large or small amounts of urine
- Voiding at more frequent intervals
- Trouble getting to the bathroom in time or feeling of urgency to void
- Painful voiding
- Difficulty starting urine stream
- Frequent dribbling of urine or feeling of bladder fullness associated with voiding small amounts of urine
- Reduced force of stream
- Accidental leakage of urine; if so, when this occurs (e.g., when coughing, laughing, or sneezing; at night; during the day)

Obtain the Medical History of Urinary Elimination Problems

- Urinary tract infections of the kidney, bladder, or urethra
- Urinary calculi
- Urinary tract surgery, such as kidney surgery, bladder surgery, prostate removal, or other surgical procedures that alter urinary routes (e.g., ureterostomy)
- Cardiovascular disease, such as hypertension or heart disease
- Chronic diseases that alter urinary characteristics or impair urinary function, such as diabetes mellitus, neurologic disease (e.g., multiple sclerosis), and cancer

Assess the Volume and Characteristics of the Client's Urine

- Time when the client last voided and the amount (Volumes of less than 30 mL or more than 500 mL per hour must be reported immediately.)
- Dark, cloudy, or discolored urine
- Presence of mucous plugs
- Offensive odor

Determine Factors Influencing Urinary Elimination

- *Medications.* Any medications that could increase urinary output (e.g., diuretics) or cause retention of urine (e.g., anticholinergic-antispasmodic drugs, antidepressant-antipsychotic drugs, antiparkinsonism drugs, antihistamines, antihypertensives) or that may discolor urine (e.g., multivitamins, phenytoin, phenothiazines). Note specific medication and dosage.
- *Fluid intake.* Amount and kind of fluid taken each day (e.g., six glasses of water, three cups of coffee, two cola drinks with or without caffeine).
- *Environmental factors.* Any problems with toileting (mobility, dexterity with clothing, toilet seat too low, facility without grab bar).
- *Presence of long-term catheter.* How the client cares for the catheter, any discomfort with it or other problems, and how the nurse can help manage it.
- *Diagnostic procedures.* Recent procedures, such as cystoscopy or spinal anesthetic.

Determine the Presence of Pain

- *Bladder pain.* Pain over the suprapubic region
- *Kidney or flank pain.* Pain between ribs and ilium, which may spread to the abdomen and be associated with nausea and vomiting, or pain at the costovertebral angle, which may radiate to the umbilicus
- *Ureteral pain.* Pain in the back, which may radiate to abdomen, upper thigh, testes, or labia

Review Data from Diagnostic Tests and Examinations

- pH under 4.5 or over 8
- Specific gravity under 1.010 or over 1.025
- Presence of glucose or acetone
- Presence of occult or visible blood
- Presence of protein, urobilinogen, or nitrite
- Presence of microorganisms
- Presence of obstructions
- Blood serum: blood urea nitrogen, creatinine, sodium, potassium

Urinary Catheterization

- Determine whether the amount of urine drained is to be limited.
- Use strict aseptic technique.
- For a retention catheter, test the balloon before insertion to see that it is intact.
- Lubricate the insertion tip of the catheter.
- Obtain assistance for a client who needs help to maintain the required position.
- For females: Clean the perineal area, keeping the labia apart once the meatus is cleaned.
- For males: Retract the foreskin of an uncircumcised client, and keep it back during the catheterization. Lift the penis perpendicular to the body before catheterization.
- Pick up and insert the catheter with your uncontaminated, sterile, gloved hand.
- Do not force a catheter beyond a major resistance.
- Before inflating the balloon of the retention catheter, insert the catheter an additional 2.5 to 5 cm (1 to 2 in.) beyond the point at which urine began to flow.
- Inflate the balloon with no more fluid than the balloon size indicates.
- After balloon inflation, apply slight tension on the catheter to check that the balloon is well anchored in

the bladder; then move the catheter slightly back into the bladder.

- Tape the catheter to the client appropriately.
- Assess the amount, color, and clarity of the urine.
- Make sure the drainage system allows free flow of urine and is well sealed or closed.

Removing a Retention Catheter

- Wear gloves.
- Deflate the balloon completely before removing it from the urethra.
- Observe the intactness of the catheter.
- Measure the urine in the drainage bag.
- Assess the frequency and amount of urine voided after catheter removal.

Special Care for Elders

The following conditions are etiologic factors in problems with urinary elimination in elders:

- Many older men have enlarged prostate glands, which can cause retention and incontinence of urine.
- Women past menopause have decreased estrogen, which results in a decrease in perineal tone and support of bladder, vagina, and supporting tissues. This often results in urgency and stress incontinence and can even increase the incidence of urinary tract infections.
- Increased stiffness and pain in joints, previous joint surgery, and neuromuscular problems can impair mobility and often make it difficult to get to the bathroom.
- Cognitive impairment, such as in dementia, often prevents the person from understanding the need to urinate and the actions needed to perform the activity. The following interventions may improve these conditions:
  - Medications or surgery to relieve obstructions in men and strengthen support in the urogenital area in women
  - Behavioral training for better bladder control

- Providing safe, easy access to the bathroom or bedside commode, whether at home or in an institution; making sure the room is well lit, environment is safe, and the proper assistive devices are within reach (such as walkers, canes)
- Habit training, such as taking the person to the bathroom at a regular, scheduled time can often work very well with cognitively impaired persons
- When catheterizing an elder, be very attentive to problems of limited movement, especially in the hips. Arthritis or previous hip or knee surgery may limit the client's movement and cause discomfort. Modify the position as needed to perform the procedure safely and comfortably. For women, obtain the assistance of another nurse to flex and hold client's knees and hips as necessary or place her in a modified Sims' position.

6. Fecal Elimination

Assess to Determine

- *Defecation pattern.* What are the frequency and time of day of the client's defecation? Has this pattern changed recently? Does it ever change? If so, does the client know what factors affect it?
- *Behavioral patterns.* The client's use of laxatives, fluids, and exercise to maintain the normal defecation pattern? What routines does the client follow to maintain the usual defecation pattern (e.g., prune juice with breakfast)?
- *Diet.* What foods does the client believe affect defecation? What foods does the client typically eat? What food does the client always avoid? Does the client take meals at regular times?
- *Fluid intake.* What amount and kind of fluid does the client take each day (e.g., four glasses of water, two cups of coffee)?
- *Exercise.* What is the client's usual daily exercise pattern? Obtain specific details; avoid asking whether the client's exercise is sufficient because people's ideas of what is sufficient differ.

- *Use of elimination aids.* What routines does the client follow to maintain usual defecation pattern? Does the client use natural aids (e.g., specific foods or fluids), laxatives, or enemas to maintain elimination?

- *Medications.* Has the client taken any medications that could affect the gastrointestinal tract (e.g., iron supplements, antihistamines in cold preparations, antacids, narcotic analgesics)?

- *Pertinent illness or surgery.* Has the client had any surgery or illness that affects the intestinal tract? Are any ostomies (e.g., colostomy or ileostomy) present?

Assess the Client's

- *Vital signs* (pulse, respirations, and blood pressure) for baseline data, particularly before administering enemas or digitally removing a fecal impaction.

- *Abdominal distention.* Distention appears as an overall outward protuberance of the abdomen, with the skin appearing tight and tense. When palpated, the abdomen feels firm. Measure a distended abdomen at the level of the umbilicus by placing a tape measure around the body. Repeated measurements indicate whether the distention is increasing or decreasing.

- *Bowel sounds.* Auscultate all four abdominal quadrants for 5 to 15 seconds to determine the degree of activity or frequency of sounds.

- *Consistency and color of feces.* Normal feces are brown and formed but soft and moist. Note color of feces. For example, black, tarry feces may indicate the presence of blood from the stomach or small intestine; acholic (pale) feces usually indicate the absence of bile; and green or orange stools may indicate the presence of an intestinal infection. Food may also affect the color of feces; for example, beets can color stool red or sometimes green. Medications, too, can alter the color of feces; iron, for example, can make stool black.

- *Presence of constipation, diarrhea, or fecal incontinence.*
- *Perianal region and anus.* Inspect these areas for discoloration, inflammations, scars, lesions, fissures, fistulas, or hemorrhoids. Note the color, size, location, and consistency of any lesion.
- *Presence of abdominal or rectal pain.*
- *Presence of flatulence and signs associated with flatulence,* such as eructations (burping) and their frequency and the passage of flatus by the rectum. Also assess respiratory rate. Flatulence can cause pressure on the diaphragm, resulting in difficult respirations.

Identify Clients at Risk for Developing Fecal Elimination Problems

- Clients who have insufficient fluid or roughage in the diet
- Clients who do not exercise sufficiently
- Clients who use constipating medications
- Clients who ingest excessive gas-forming foods

Administering an Enema
For All Enemas

- Determine the type and purpose of the enema and whether a primary care provider's order is required.
- Position the client appropriately.
- Wear clean gloves.
- Assess the returns.

Cleansing Enema

- Use the correct type, amount, and temperature of solution.
- To remove air, flush the tubing before administering the enema.
- Lubricate the rectal tube before insertion.
- Direct the insertion tube toward the client's umbilicus.
- Ask the client to take a deep breath during tube insertion.

- Hold the solution container at the correct height.
- Administer the solution slowly, and start and stop the flow of solution temporarily if the client complains of cramping.

Retention Enema

- Instruct client to try to retain the enema at least 30 minutes.

Special Care for Elders

- Elders may fatigue easily.
- Elders may be more susceptible to fluid and electrolyte imbalances. Use tap water enemas with great caution.
- Monitor the client's tolerance during the procedure, watching for vagal episodes and dysrhythmias.
- Protect elders' skin from prolonged exposure to moisture.
- Assist elders with perineal care as indicated.

7. Pressure Areas
Assess to Determine

- The client's need for supportive devices, such as pillows, rolled or folded towels, foam supports, footboard, hand rolls, wrist splints, or sandbags by assessing the following in the client:

  - *Adipose tissue.* A client who has ample adipose tissue generally requires less support and cushioning than the emaciated person does while in a back-lying position, but greater support to maintain a lateral position.

  - *Skeletal structure.* Both the amount and the type of support needed vary according to the individual's skeletal structure. A person with a marked lumbar lordosis requires more lumbar support than one with a slight lumbar curvature.

  - *Health status.* A person who has flaccid or spastic paralysis requires supportive devices. The support differs with the client's specific health status.

- *Discomfort.* A person who experiences pain during movement requires more support during movement than one who can move without pain. A person who is unconscious is unable to indicate discomfort and needs appropriate support and change of position at least every 2 hours.

- *Skin condition.* People who have nutritional problems or impaired circulation require more cushioning of the pressure points to prevent skin breakdown than do healthy people.

- *Ability to move.* People who can move in bed can change position frequently. The client who is unable to move (e.g., the unconscious client) requires support and positioning.

- *Hydration.* Dehydrated clients are at greater risk of pressure ulcer formation than well-hydrated clients and therefore need more support under pressure areas.

Assess the Client's

- Strength and ability to move before the change of position, and obtain assistance as required. Appropriate assistance reduces the risk of muscle strain and body injury to both the client and nurse.

- Pressure areas of the body for any pale or reddened spots. This discoloration, which can be caused by impaired blood circulation to the area, should disappear in a few minutes when pressure relief restores circulation. See Figure 3–1 for the location of pressure areas.

- Pressure areas of the body for abrasions and excoriations. An abrasion (wearing away of the skin) can occur when skin rubs against a sheet, such as when the client is pulled. Excoriations (loss of superficial layers of the skin) can occur when the skin has prolonged contact with body secretions or excretions, or with dampness in skinfolds.

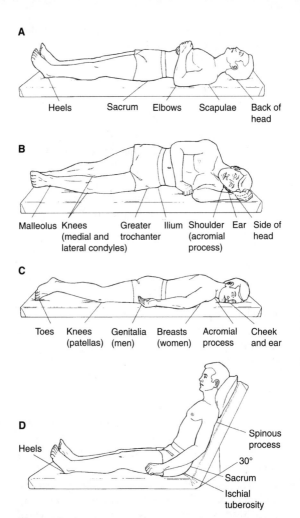

Figure 3–1 ■ Body pressure areas in **A**, supine position; **B**, lateral position; **C**, prone position; **D**, Fowler's position.

- Stage of pressure ulcers if present. The four stages of pressure ulcers are described as follows (National Pressure Ulcer Advisory Panel, 2007):

  Stage I: Nonblanchable erythema signaling potential ulceration

  Stage II: Abrasion, blister, or shallow crater involving the epidermis and possibly the dermis

  Stage III: Full-thickness skin extending through the subcutaneous layer to the fascia

  Stage IV: Tissue necrosis and damage involving muscle, bone, or supporting structures

Palpate (with Warm Hands)

- The surface temperature of the skin over pressure areas. Normally, the temperature is the same as that of the surrounding skin. Increased temperature is abnormal and may be due to inflammation or blood trapped in the area. A decreased temperature indicates impaired circulation.

- Over bony prominences and dependent body areas for the presence of edema. Edema feels spongy on palpation.

Treating Pressure Ulcers

- Minimize direct pressure on the ulcer. Reposition the client at least every 2 hours. Make a schedule, and record position changes on the client's chart.

- Reduce friction on intact skin by using proper lifting and moving techniques.

- Reduce shearing force by keeping the head of the bed flat or elevated to a maximum of 30 degrees, unless contraindicated by the client's condition.

- Teach the client to move, even if only slightly, to relieve pressure.

- Encourage ambulation or sitting in a wheelchair as the client's condition permits.

- Provide range-of-motion exercises as the client's condition permits.
- Clean the pressure ulcer daily. Use a method consistent with the stage of the ulcer and agency protocol.
- Dress the ulcer using surgical asepsis. Refrain from using antiseptics, such as alcohol, that are vasoconstrictors and reduce blood flow to the area.

Special Care for Elders

- If the client cannot keep weight off the pressure ulcer, use pressure-relieving devices, such as foam gel pads or mattresses or specialty beds.

- Hold wrinkled skin taut during application of a transparent dressing. Obtain assistance if needed.

- Skin is more fragile and can easily tear with removal of tape (especially adhesive tape). Use paper tape and tape remover as indicated, keeping tape use to the minimum required. Use extreme caution during tape removal.

- Elders in long-term care facilities often have immobility, malnutrition, and incontinence—all of which increase the risk for development of skin breakdown.

- Skin breakdown can occur as quickly as within 2 hours, so assessments should be done with each repositioning of the client.

- A thorough assessment of a client's heels should be done every shift. The skin can break down quickly from friction of movement in bed. (See Table 3–1 for pressure ulcer dressings.)

References

National Pressure Ulcer Advisory Panel. (2007). *Pressure Ulcer Stages*. Washington D.C.: Author. Retrieved March 1, 2007, from http://www.npuap.org/documents/ NPUAP2007_PU_Def_and_Descriptions.pdf.

Table 3-1 Selected Types of Wound Dressings

Dressing	Description	Purpose	Indications
Transparent film	Adhesive plastic, semipermeable, nonabsorbent dressings allow exchange of oxygen between the atmosphere and wound bed. Impermeable to bacteria and water.	Protection against contamination and friction; maintain a clean, moist surface that facilitates cellular migration; provide insulation by preventing fluid evaporation; facilitate wound assessment	Intravenous dressing Central line dressing Superficial wounds Pressure ulcers stage I
Impregnated nonadherent	Woven or nonwoven cotton or synthetic materials impregnated with petrolatum, saline, zinc-saline, antimicrobials, or other agents. Require secondary dressings to secure them in place, retain moisture, and provide wound protection.	Cover, soothe, and protect partial- and full-thickness wounds without exudate	Postoperative dressing over staple/sutures Superficial burns
Hydrocolloids	Waterproof adhesive wafers, pastes, or powders. Inner adhesive layer has particles that absorb exudates and form a hydrated gel over the wound; outer film provides an occlusive seal.	Absorb exudate; produce a moist environment that facilitates healing but does not cause maceration of surrounding skin; protect the wound from bacterial contamination, foreign debris, and urine or feces; and prevent shearing	Pressure ulcers stage II–IV Autolytic débridement of eschar Partial thickness wounds

(continued)

Table 3–1 Selected Types of Wound Dressings *(continued)*

Dressing	Description	Purpose	Indications
Clear absorbent acrylic dressing	Transparent absorbent wafer. Acrylic layer absorbs exudates and evaporates the excess off the transparent membrane.	Maintains a transparent membrane for easy wound bed assessment, provides bacterial and sharing protection; maintains moist wound healing; can be used with alginates to provide packing to deeper wound beds	Pressure ulcers
Skin tears
Venous stasis ulcers
Surgical wounds
Wounds undergoing chemical débridement agents
Hydrogels	Glycerin- or water-based nonadhesive jellylike sheets, granules, or gels are oxygen-permeable, unless covered by a plastic film. Require secondary occlusive dressing.	Liquefy necrotic tissue or slough, rehydrate the wound bed, and fill in dead space	Pressure ulcers
Skin tears
Partial-thickness wounds

| Polyurethane foams | Nonadherent hydrocolloid dressings. Require secondary dressings to obtain an occlusive environment. Surrounding skin must be protected to prevent maceration. | Absorb up to heavy amounts of exudate; provide and maintain moist wound healing | Light to highly exudating wounds
Pressure ulcers
Skin tears
Venous stasis ulcers
Surgical wounds
Wounds undergoing chemical débridement agents |
| Alginates (exudate absorbers) | Nonadherent dressings of powder, beads or granules, ropes, sheets, or paste conform to the wound surface and absorb up to 20 times their weight in exudate. Require a secondary dressing. | Provide moist wound surface by interacting with exudate to form a gelatinous mass; absorb exudate; eliminate dead space or pack wounds; support débridement | Pressure ulcers
Skin tears
Venous stasis ulcers
Surgical wounds
Wounds undergoing chemical débridement agents |

B. Clinical Guidelines   103

8. Healing Wounds

Assess to Determine

Appearance

- Inspect color of wound and surrounding area and approximation of wound edges.

Size

- Note size and location of dehiscence, if present. For wounds healing by secondary intention, measure the length, width, and depth in centimeters.

Drainage

- Observe location, color, consistency, odor, and degree of saturation of dressings. Note number of gauzes saturated or diameter of drainage on gauze.

Swelling

- Wearing sterile gloves, palpate wound edges for tension and tautness of tissues; minimal to moderate swelling is normal in early stages of wound healing.

Pain

- Expect severe to moderate postoperative pain for 3 to 5 days; persistent severe pain or sudden onset of severe pain may indicate internal hemorrhaging or infection.

Drains or Tubes

- Inspect drain security and placement, amount and character of drainage, and functioning of collecting apparatus, if present.

Changing a Dry Sterile Dressing

- Support the adjacent skin when removing adhesive tape.
- Pull tape toward the wound rather than away from it.
- Wear disposable gloves when removing moist outer dressings.
- Use sterile forceps or gloves to remove inner dressings.
- Support a drain appropriately when removing dressings.

- Use separate sterile forceps to clean and dress the wound.
- Use a separate swab for each cleaning stroke.
- Clean the wound from the least contaminated to the most contaminated area.
- Clean a drain site after the incision.
- Dry the wound appropriately.
- Assess the wound appearance and drainage accurately.
- Apply sufficient dressings to cover the wound and absorb drainage.
- Secure the dressing with adhesive tape or wrapping gauze, as appropriate.

Applying Damp-to-Damp Dressings

- Before applying the dressing, medicate the client for pain as indicated.
- Maintain asepsis.
- Verify the ordered solution, and check agency policy about cleaning the wound.
- Assess the wound appearance and drainage.
- Thoroughly saturate the mesh gauze with solution, and then wring out excess moisture.
- Make sure all depressions and grooves of the wound are packed with the gauze.
- Cover the damp dressings appropriately. Do not apply an airtight occlusive covering.
- To keep the gauze damp, change or remoisten with saline frequently.
- Although gauze is much less expensive than advanced dressings (e.g., polymers, alginates, collagens), the cost per week can be higher due to the number of dressing changes required.

Special Care for Elders

- Elders may need extra support during dressing changes, especially if arthritis, contractures, or tremors are present.

- Avoid constricting the client's circulation with a tight bandage or binder. Observe skin and bony prominences frequently for signs of impaired circulation. The risk for skin breakdown increases with age.

9. Postoperative Period
Assess to Determine

- *Vital signs: pulse, respirations, and blood pressure.* Compare results with data from the recovery room and preoperative baseline data. Many hospitals have postoperative routines for regular assessment of clients. In some agencies, assessments are made every 15 minutes until vital signs stabilize, every hour thereafter the same day, and every 4 hours for the next 2 days. Body temperature is usually assessed every 4 hours for the first few days. *It is vital that the assessments be made as frequently as the person's condition requires.* An elevated temperature, along with other signs, can indicate infection of the respiratory tract, urinary tract, or incision. A rapid, weak pulse and increased respiratory rate along with other signs can indicate infection, hemorrhage, or shock. A lowered blood pressure along with other signs can indicate hemorrhage, shock, or pulmonary embolism.

- *Skin color and temperature.* The color of the lips and nail beds is an indicator of tissue perfusion (passage of blood through the capillaries). Pale, cyanotic, cool, and moist skin may be a sign of circulatory problems.

- *Level of consciousness.* During the early postoperative period, most clients are conscious but drowsy.

- *Bleeding.* Inspect the dressings for bleeding, and inspect the bedclothes underneath the client for pooled blood. When dressings are changed, inspect the wound for signs of localized infection.

- *Intravenous infusion.* Observe the type of solution, the amount in the bottle, the drip rate, and the venipuncture site. Determine additional solutions ordered.

- *Patency of drainage tubes*. Note also the amount, color, consistency, and character of the drainage.

- *Fluid balance*. Measure the client's fluid intake and output for at least 2 days or until fluid balance is stable without an intravenous infusion.

- *Pain or discomfort and when the client last received an analgesic*. Note the location and type of pain, and determine the cause. Pain is usually greatest 12 to 36 hours after surgery, decreasing on the second or third day. Analgesics are usually administered every 3 or 4 hours the first day, and by the third day most clients require only oral analgesics. Signs of acute pain include pallor, perspiration, tension, and reluctance to perform deep-breathing and coughing exercises or to move or ambulate.

- *Any difficulties with voiding and/or bladder distention.*

- *Return of peristalsis*. Auscultate the client's abdomen to confirm the return of peristalsis. Note the passage of flatus and stool.

- *Tolerance of food and fluids ingested.*

Determine Clinical Signs of Postoperative Complications

- *Pneumonia*: Elevated temperature, cough, expectoration of blood-tinged or purulent sputum, dyspnea, chest pain.

- *Atelectasis*: Marked dyspnea, cyanosis, pleural pain, tachycardia, increased respiratory rate, fever, productive cough, auscultatory crackling sounds.

- *Pulmonary embolism*: Sudden chest pain, shortness of breath, cyanosis, shock (tachycardia, low blood pressure).

- *Thrombophlebitis*: Aching, cramping pain; affected area is swollen, red, and hot to touch; vein feels hard; discomfort in calf when foot is dorsiflexed or when client walks (Homans' sign).

- *Thrombus or embolus*: Same as for pulmonary embolism; if lodged in heart or brain, assess cardiac or neurologic signs.
- *Urinary retention*: Fluid intake larger than output, inability to void or frequent voiding of small amounts, bladder distention, suprapubic discomfort, restlessness, bladder palpable above the pubic symphysis.
- *Urinary infection*: Burning sensation when voiding, urgency, cloudy urine, lower abdominal pain.
- *Constipation*: Absence of stool elimination, abdominal distention, and discomfort.
- *Tympanites*: Obvious abdominal distention, abdominal discomfort (gas pains), absence of bowel sounds.
- *Wound infection*: Purulent exudate, redness, tenderness, elevated body temperature, wound odor.
- *Wound dehiscence*: Increased incision drainage; tissues underlying skin become visible along parts of the incision.
- *Wound evisceration*: Opening of incision and visible protrusion of organs.

Managing Gastrointestinal Suction

- Confirm the placement of the nasogastric tube before establishing suction.
- Place an air vent appropriately, and maintain its patency by injecting air.
- Test the functioning of the suction system before connecting it.
- Prevent kinks or blockages in the tubing.
- Keep all connections well sealed.
- Inspect the flow of gastric secretions into the drainage bottle.
- Clean the nares around the nasogastric tube at least every 3 hours.
- Provide mouth care.

Irrigations

- Obtain the physician's order if needed.

- Confirm the placement of the tube before irrigation.
- Reconnect the tube, and attach it to suction after irrigating.
- Assess the amount and character of the drainage, client comfort, and abdominal distention.

Preventing Infections in the Home

- Wash your hands before handling foods, before eating, after toileting, before and after any required home care treatment, and after touching any body substances (e.g., wound drainage).
- Keep your fingernails short, clean, and well manicured to eliminate rough edges or hangnails, which can harbor microorganisms.
- Do not share personal care items: toothbrush, washcloths, and towels.
- Wash raw fruits and vegetables before eating them.
- Refrigerate all opened and nonpackaged foods.
- Clean used equipment (e.g., emesis basin) with soap and water, and disinfect it with a chlorine bleach solution.
- Place contaminated dressings and other disposable items containing body fluids in moisture-proof plastic bags.
- Put used needles in a puncture-resistant container with a screw-top lid. Label so as not to discard in the garbage.
- Clean obviously soiled linen separately from other laundry. Rinse in cold water, wash in hot water if possible, and add a cup of bleach or Lysol to the wash.
- Avoid coughing, sneezing, or breathing directly on others. Cover the mouth and nose to prevent the transmission of airborne microorganisms.
- Be aware of any signs or symptoms of an infection, and report these immediately to your health care contact person.
- Maintain a sufficient fluid intake to promote urine production and output. This helps flush the bladder and urethra of microorganisms.

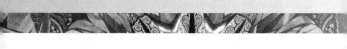

C. Teaching and Learning Guidelines

Teaching is a process designed to produce specific learning. The teaching and learning process involves dynamic interaction between the teacher and the learner. For teaching to be effective, trust must be established between the teacher and the learner, and communication must be open. Teaching is a five-step process analogous to the nursing process:

1. Collect data; analyze client's learning strengths and deficits.
2. Make educational diagnoses.
3. Prepare teaching plan.
4. Implement teaching plan.
5. Evaluate client learning (effectiveness of teaching process).

Nurses teach in a variety of ways and settings. Teaching may be planned, as in preoperative teaching. Teaching may also result during an interaction with a client. For example, when caring for a postoperative client, you find the client tense and in pain. Although the client has patient-controlled analgesia, you assess that the client does not understand how to use the pump. As part of your professional responsibilities, you must first make the client comfortable by administering the appropriate pain medicine and then teach the client how to use the patient-controlled analgesia device.

Teaching can occur in many settings. In the hospital, teaching may be part of your daily client care. It may also be more formal, as in childbirth preparation classes or diabetes education classes. Teaching is a large part of home health and community health nursing. Teaching occurs in any location where nurses interact with clients.

When planning your client teaching, consider the following points:

- Learning requires energy and the ability to concentrate. Extreme anxiety or such physiologic factors as pain or sleep deprivation make it difficult for the client to learn. The nurse needs to consider the client's physical condition. The client who has been medicated for pain may or may not be ready for teaching. If the client is groggy from the medication, defer teaching; if, however, the pain medication has allowed the client to relax and become alert, this may be a good time to conduct a teaching session.

- Motivation is a powerful facilitator of learning. Clients who understand why they need to learn and who recognize the benefit of this knowledge are more likely to succeed. For example, the hazards of smoking are well known. Telling clients that quitting the habit will improve their health may not be sufficient; you must find out what is important to them so that the teaching is based on their learning needs, not yours.

- To maximize learning, create the best learning environment. It is often difficult to teach in a crowded hospital room. Roommates may have visitors or the television may be on, and privacy may not be possible. Attempt to modify the environment to promote learning. Plan to teach during quiet hours and when the client is comfortable and alert. Sometimes it is best to take the client to a quiet conference room.

- Establish rapport with the client before you begin instruction. Find out who the client is and what the client already knows. Build on the client's prior knowledge.

- Present your teaching in a form that the client can understand. Language and cultural differences may affect learning. For the client who speaks a different language, arrange translator services. Be careful when using family or support system members as translators. If it is important for family members to be part of the learning process, avoid asking them to act as translators; they may be so busy translating that they cannot take in the information you present.

- Honor cultural differences. To establish rapport with the client and family, approach them with respect. Attempt to learn about the client's beliefs and values. Teaching that is in violation of cultural beliefs has little likelihood of succeeding. For more information on cultural issues, see Chapter 18 of *Fundamentals of Nursing*.

- Be certain to speak at the level the client can understand. Health care workers often speak in jargon. For example, a client may not understand what you mean when you say, "I'm going to straight cath you in order to get a sterile urine for C&S." You will need to explain this in terms with which the client is familiar and at the level that is appropriate for the client.

- Know your client. Choose your teaching strategy based on the client. Good teaching begins with client assessment. Determine what type of learner the client is, and orient your teaching according to this assessment. Is the client an auditory learner? If so, arrange a quiet time to talk. Is the client a visual learner? If so, discussion is not the best teaching strategy for this client. Instead, try drawings and pictures or videotapes. Is the client a hands-on learner, or is the material best presented in this fashion? Teaching a client how to self-administer an injection cannot be accomplished by merely talking about the technique. This type of teaching is best conducted by allowing the client to handle the syringe and medication.

- When teaching home care strategies, make sure you acquire adequate information about the home environment. Take the time to learn about the client so that the teaching is tailored to the client's situation. Suppose you are the hospital nurse caring for a client who has fallen and broken her hip. She has had surgery, and you are preparing her for discharge home. If the client is using a walker, can she get into a narrow bathroom with her walker? If she cannot yet negotiate stairs, how will she manage at home if the bedroom and bath are upstairs and the kitchen downstairs? Interview the client so that your teaching can be geared to her situation. Maybe she needs a home health aide. You will not know if you do not ask, and if you do not ask, the client may be back in the hospital with further problems.

- Make sure you are teaching the right person. Suppose, for example, that a beginning nursing student is caring for a newly diagnosed client with diabetes and gives him detailed instruction on modifying his diet. However, when making a home visit, the nurse finds that none of this information is being used. The teaching had been directed to the wrong person because, as the client then informs the nurse, he does not do the shopping or the cooking. The nurse had failed to include the right person in her teaching. She should have asked the client's partner to participate in the diet instruction.

- Provide frequent feedback. Praise clients for what they have done well, and continue to work on areas that need improvement.

To summarize, effective teaching:
- Holds the learner's interest.
- Fosters a positive self-concept in the learner; learner believes learning is probable.
- Supports the learner with positive reinforcement.
- Makes partners of the learner and the teacher.
- Is accurate and current.
- Is appropriate for the learner's age, condition, and abilities.
- Is optimistic, positive, and nonthreatening.

Special Care for Elders
Teaching and Learning

Elders often have chronic illnesses that require multiple treatments and/or medications. Health teaching focuses on the same areas as with other ages—health and wellness promotion and prevention of illness and accidents—but often the needs are greatest in learning to live with conditions that they have and to maintain optimal health and functioning. For elders to be motivated to learn, the material must be practical and have meaning for them individually, especially if the information is new to them. Special considerations in teaching elders are as follows:

- Make health promotion a priority need and include the following areas:
  - Exercise
  - Nutrition
  - Safety habits
  - Regular health check-ups
  - Understanding of medications
- Set achievable goals; involve the client and family.
- If using visual aids, use large print and contrasting colors.
- Increase time for teaching, allow for rest periods.
- Repeat information if necessary.
- Use return demonstrations with psychomotor skills, such as teaching someone how to do insulin injections.
- Determine where elders obtain most of their health information (newspapers, magazines, television).
- Use examples that they can relate to in their daily life.
- Be aware of sensory deficits, such as hearing and vision.
- Use the setting where the individual is most comfortable—either a group or one-on-one setting.
- If noncompliance is a problem, investigate the cause—it could be due to lack of finances, transportation problems, or poor access to medical care.

Elders come with a lifetime of experiences and learned knowledge of their own. Respect this, and always have them use their strengths to work with any problems. Positive reinforcement and ongoing evaluation of what has been taught are important factors in effective health teaching with elders.

References

Hayes, K. (2005). Designing written medication instructions. *Journal of Gerontological Nursing, 31*(5), 5–10.

Stanley, M., Blair, K., & Beare, P. G. (2005). *Gerontological nursing: Promoting successful aging with older adults*, 3rd ed. (pp. 67–75). Philadelphia: F. A. Davis Co.

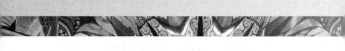

D. MEDICATIONS

Proper management of client medications is essential to safe patient care. A survey on use of drugs and medications, any allergies, or reports of problems with medications should be part of every nursing history. Safety consciousness should be uppermost in your mind when you administer medications. Always practice the "rights" for accurate medication administration:

- Right client
- Right medication
- Right dose
- Right time
- Right route
- Right documentation
- Right client education
- Right assessment
- Right evaluation
- Right to refuse

Check each medication thoroughly, and check the accuracy of the medication administration record with the physician's order. A medication order must be complete. It must contain the client's name, the date, the medication, dose, route, method of administration, and signature of the prescriber. If any section of the order is unclear, difficult to read, or missing, contact the physician or advanced practice nurse. See Chapter 35 of *Fundamentals of Nursing* for a thorough discussion of medications, and remember, client safety must come first!

Check the medication against the order to be certain you are using the right medication. Many medications have similar names. Often a medication may be ordered in a trade name but be available in a generic form. Consult a drug guide to check for equivalency. With newer medications, you may need to consult a pharmacist for this type of information. After you have completed your preparation of the medication, check again for accuracy before you administer the medication to the client. Identify the client before administering any medication. Check the client's name band against the medication administration record. If the name band is missing, ask the client to identify himself or herself, or ask another nurse to verify the client's identity. The Joint Commission on Accreditation of Healthcare Organizations requires a nurse to use at least two client identifiers whenever administering medications. Neither identifier can be the client's room number. Acceptable identifiers may be the person's name, assigned identification number, telephone number, photograph, or other person-specific identifier.

Your responsibility does not end once you administer the medication. A record must be kept of all medications administered. Promptly chart them after you administer them. When you get busy, it is tempting to postpone your charting. However, you run the risk that your preceptor will repeat the administration. Likewise, never chart a medication before giving it. When you chart, you are stating that you have prepared the medication and that the client has taken it. Too many things can go wrong if you prechart—the client may refuse, the client may be away from the unit at the prescribed time, or the client may even expire. Always chart that you have given the medication only after you have given it.

- Nurses who administer medications are responsible for their own actions. Question any order that you consider incorrect.

- Be knowledgeable about the medications you administer.

- Federal laws govern the uses of narcotics and barbiturates. Keep these medications in a locked place.

- Use only medications that are in a clearly labeled container.

- Return liquid medications that are cloudy or have changed color to the pharmacy.

- Do not leave medication at the bedside, with certain exceptions (e.g., nitroglycerin). Determine agency policy.

- If a client vomits after taking an oral medication, report this to the nurse in charge.

- Take special precautions when administering certain medications; for example, have another nurse check the dosages of anticoagulants, insulin, and certain intravenous preparations.

- Most hospitals require new orders from the physician for the client's postsurgery care.

- When a medication is omitted for any reason, record the fact together with the reason.

- When a medication error is made, report it immediately to the nurse in charge.

Table 3–2 includes common abbreviations used in medication orders. Table 3–3 includes unacceptable abbreviations.

Table 3–2 Common Abbreviations Used in Medication Orders

Abbreviation	Explanation	Example of Administration Time
ac	before meals	0700, 1100, and 1700 hrs
ad lib	freely, as desired	
bid	twice a day	0900 and 2100 hrs
$\bar{c}$	with	
cap	capsule	
elix	elixir	
g (G)	gram	
gr	grain	
gtt	drop	
h	an hour	
hs	at bedtime	

Table 3–2 Common Abbreviations Used in Medication Orders

Abbreviation	Explanation	Example of Administration Time
IM	intramuscular	
IV	intravenous	
m	minim	
mg	milligram	
mL (ml)	milliliter	
OD	right eye	
OS	left eye	
OU	both eyes	
pc	after meals	0900, 1300, and 1900 hrs
po	by mouth	
prn	when needed	
q	every	
QAM	every morning	1000 hrs
Rx	take, prescription	
s ($\bar{s}$)	without	
sig (s)	label	
ss ($\overline{ss}$)	one-half	
sup (supp)	suppository	
susp	suspension	
tid	three times a day	1000, 1400, and 1800 hrs

Table 3–3 Unacceptable Abbreviations—"Do Not Use" List

Abbreviation	Potential Problem	Use Instead
U (unit)	Mistaken for "0" (zero), the number "4" (four), or "cc"	Write "unit"
IU (international unit)	Mistaken for IV (intravenous) or the number 10 (ten)	Write "International Unit"
Q.D., QD, q.d., qd (daily)	Mistaken for each other	Write "daily"
Q.O.D., QOD, q.o.d., qod (every other day)	Period after the "Q" mistaken for "I" and the "O" mistaken for "I"	Write "every other day"
Trailing zero (X.0 mg)	Decimal point is missed	Write X mg
Lack of leading zero (.X mg)	Decimal point is missed	Write 0.X mg

Abbreviation	Potential Problem	Use Instead
MS	Can mean morphine sulfate or magnesium sulfate	Write "morphine sulfate"
MSO$_4$ and MgSO$_4$	Can mean morphine sulfate or magnesium sulfate	Write "magnesium sulfate"

For Possible Future Inclusion in the Official "Do Not Use" List

> (greater than)	Misinterpreted as the number "7" (seven) or the letter "L"	Write "greater than"
< (less than)	Confused for one another	Write "less than"
Abbreviations for drug names	Misinterpreted due to similar abbreviations for multiple drugs	Write drug names in full
Apothecary units	Unfamiliar to many practitioners	Use metric units
	Confused with metric units	
@	Mistaken for the number "2" (two)	Write "at"
cc	Mistaken for "U" (units) when poorly written	Write "mL" or "milliliters"
μg	Mistaken for mg (milligrams), resulting in 1000-fold overdose	Write "mcg" or "micrograms"

Others to Consider

TIW (three times a week)	Has been misinterpreted as "two times a week" or "three times a day," resulting in misdosing	Write "three times weekly"
AS (left ear) AD (right ear) AU (both ears)	Mistaken for "OS" (left eye), "OD" (either "overdose" or "optic density"), and "OU" ("each eye" or "both eyes")	Write "left ear," "right ear," or "both ears," as appropriate
HS	Has been used to indicate "half strength" and "bedtime" or "hour of sleep"	Write out "half strength" or "at bedtime," as appropriate
SC and SQ (subcutaneous)	Have been read as "SL" (sublingual) and as "5 every hour"	Write "subq" or "subcutaneous"
D/C	Can mean either "discharge" or "discontinue"	Write "discharge" or "discontinue," as appropriate

Converting Weights and Measures Among Systems

When preparing client medications, a nurse may need to convert weights or volumes from one system to another. As an example, the pharmacy may dispense milligrams or grams of chloral hydrate, yet the nurse must administer an order that reads chloral hydrate grains viiss. To prepare the correct dose, the nurse must convert from the apothecaries' to the metric system. To give clients a useful, realistic measure for home use, the nurse may have to convert from the apothecaries' or metric system to the household system. All conversions are approximate—that is, not totally precise.

For example, a physician orders morphine gr $^1/_4$. The medication is available only in milligrams. The nurse knows that 1 mg = $^1/_{60}$ gr, or 60 mg = 1 grain. To convert the ordered dose to milligrams, the nurse calculates as follows:

$$\text{If } 1 \text{ gr} = 60 \text{ mg}$$
$$\text{Then } ^1/_4 \text{ gr } (0.25 \text{ gr}) = x \text{ mg}$$
$$\text{Cross multiply: } x = 60 \times 0.25$$
$$x = 15 \text{ mg}$$

Calculating Dosages

Several formulas can be used to calculate drug dosages. One formula uses ratios:

$$\frac{\text{dose on hand}}{\text{quantity on hand}} = \frac{\text{desired dose}}{\text{quantity desired } (x)}$$

For example, erythromycin 500 mg is ordered. It is supplied in a liquid form containing 250 mg in 5 mL. To calculate the dosage, use the formula:

$$\frac{\text{dose on hand (250 mg)}}{\text{quantity on hand (5 mL)}} = \frac{\text{desired dose (500 mg)}}{\text{quantity desired } (x \text{ mL})}$$

Then, cross-multiply:

$$250 \, x = 5 \text{ mL} \times 500 \text{ mg}$$
$$x = \frac{5 \text{ mL} \times 500 \text{ mg}}{250 \text{ mL}}$$
$$x = 10 \text{ mL}$$

Therefore, the dose ordered is 10 mL.

Another method for dosage calculation is the following:

amount to administer $(x) =$

$$\frac{\text{desired dose}}{\text{dose on hand} \times \text{quantity on hand}}$$

For example, heparin can be distributed in vials and prepared dilutions of 10,000 units per mL. If the order calls for 5000 units, the nurse can calculate using the previous formula:

$$x = \frac{5000 \text{ units}}{10,000 \text{ units}} \times 1 \,\text{mL}$$

$$x = {}^1\!/_2 \,\text{mL}$$

Therefore, the nurse injects 0.5 mL for a 5000-unit dose.

Injection Techniques

Review Figures 3–2 to 3–5 for injection sites, types of injections, and injection techniques.

Special Care for Elders

Medications

- The physiologic changes associated with aging influence medication administration and effectiveness. Examples include altered memory, less acute vision, decrease in renal function, less complete and slower absorption from the gastrointestinal tract, and decreased liver function. Many of these changes enhance the possibility of cumulative effects and toxicity.

- Elders usually require smaller dosages of drugs, especially sedatives and other central nervous system depressants.

- Elders are mature adults capable of reasoning. The nurse therefore needs to explain the reasons for and the effects of the client's medications.

- Elders may have a decreased muscle mass or muscle atrophy. A shorter needle may be needed. Assessment of appropriate injection site is critical. Absorption of medication may occur more quickly than expected.

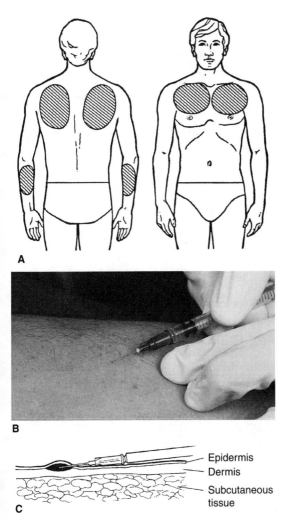

Figure 3–2 ■ A, Body sites commonly used for intradermal injections. For an intradermal injection: B, the needle enters the skin at a 15-degree angle; and C, the medication forms a bleb under the epidermis.

Epidermis
Dermis
Subcutaneous tissue

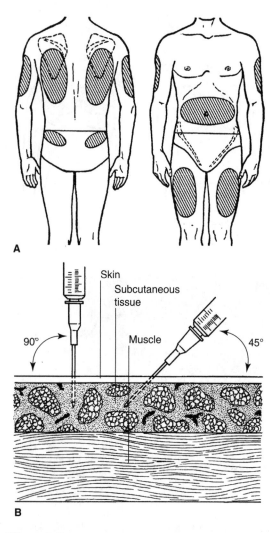

Figure 3–3 ■ **A,** Body sites commonly used for subcutaneous injections. **B,** Inserting a needle into the subcutaneous tissue using 90-degree and 45-degree angles.

Skin
Subcutaneous tissue
Muscle
90°
45°

A

B

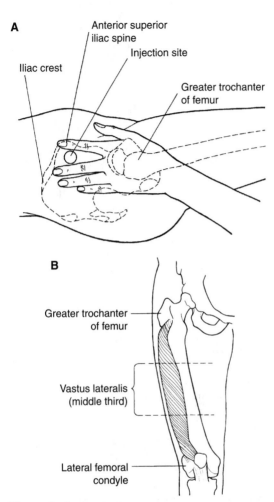

A

Iliac crest

Anterior superior
iliac spine

Injection site

Greater trochanter
of femur

B

Greater trochanter
of femur

Vastus lateralis
(middle third)

Lateral femoral
condyle

Figure 3–4 ■ Body sites commonly used for intramuscular injections. **A,** the ventrogluteal site for an intramuscular injection; **B,** the vastus lateralis site for an intramuscular injection. *(Continued)*

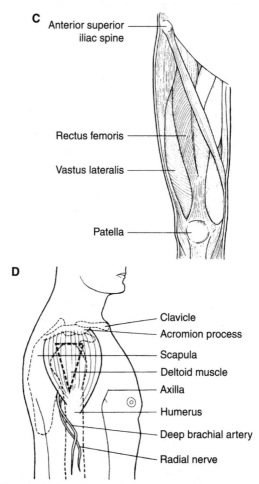

C

Anterior superior iliac spine

Rectus femoris

Vastus lateralis

Patella

D

Clavicle

Acromion process

Scapula

Deltoid muscle

Axilla

Humerus

Deep brachial artery

Radial nerve

Figure 3–4 ■ Body sites commonly used for intramuscular injections. **C,** the rectus femoris muscle of the upper right thigh, used for intramuscular injections; **D,** the deltoid muscle of the upper arm, used for intramuscular injections. *(Continued)*

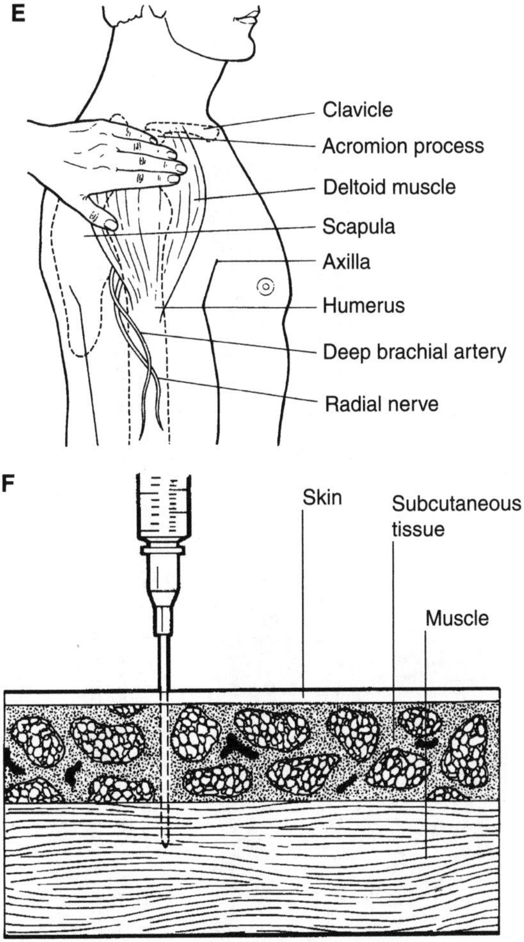
E
Clavicle
Acromion process
Deltoid muscle
Scapula
Axilla
Humerus
Deep brachial artery
Radial nerve
F
Skin
Subcutaneous
tissue
Muscle

Figure 3–4 ■ Body sites commonly used for intramuscular injections. **E,** a method of establishing the deltoid muscle for an intramuscular injection; **F,** an intramuscular needle inserted into the muscle layer.

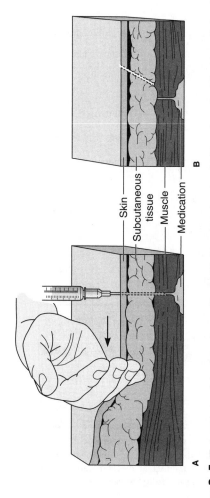

Skin

Subcutaneous
tissue

Muscle

Medication

A

B

Figure 3–5 ■ Inserting an intramuscular needle at a 90-degree angle using the Z-track method: *A*, skin pulled to the side; *B*, skin released. *Note:* When the skin returns to its normal position after the needle is withdrawn, a seal is formed over the intramuscular site. This prevents seepage of the medication into the subcutaneous tissues and subsequent discomfort.

UNIT 4

DOCUMENTATION AND EVALUATION

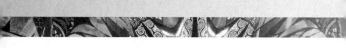

A. Charting Guidelines

Charting is a written method of conveying client information, nursing assessments and interventions, and client response to care. For a thorough discussion of documentation and reporting, review Chapter 15 of *Fundamentals of Nursing.* The following list of guidelines can help you chart accurately:

- Make sure the nursing record is stamped with the client's name before you begin writing. If using a computer, make sure it is the correct client record.

- Write legibly; print if necessary. Always write in permanent ink. Check agency policy for color of ink.

- Begin each entry with the time and date of the recording. End each entry with a signature that consists of your first initial, last name, and abbreviated title.

- Never erase or use correction fluid (Wite-Out). Cross through a mistake with a single line, write the word "mistaken entry" above it, and initial the change.

- If a blank space appears in a notation, draw a line through the blank space so that no additional information can be recorded at any other time or by any other person.

- Write your notes as soon as possible after giving nursing care.

- Be precise. State your assessments objectively. Report the client's subjective opinions by quoting directly. Avoid using words that convey judgment or inference—just state the facts.

- Chart the client's response to interventions.
- Use only commonly accepted abbreviations, symbols, and terms specified by the agency. Know the "Do Not Use" list of abbreviations (see pages 120 and 121).
- Record your teaching.
- Review your notes—are they clear and what you want to say?
- Remember that from a legal perspective, if you did not chart it, you did not do it!

Essential Client Information

The following may assist you in selecting essential client information to record. Note that you should emphasize data that denote a change in the client's health status or behavior and data that indicate a deviation from what is usually expected.

1. Any behavior changes, for example,
   - Indications of strong emotions, such as anxiety or fear
   - Marked changes in mood
   - A change in level of consciousness, such as stupor
   - Regression in relationships with family or friends
2. Any changes in physical function, such as
   - Loss of balance
   - Loss of strength
   - Difficulty hearing or seeing
3. Any physical sign or symptom that
   - Is severe, such as severe pain
   - Tends to recur or persist
   - Deviates from normal, such as elevated body temperature
   - Gets worse, such as weight loss
   - Indicates faulty health habits, such as lice on the scalp

- Is a known danger signal, such as a lump in the breast

4. Any nursing interventions provided, such as
   - Medications administered
   - Therapies
   - Activities of daily living, if agency policy dictates
   - Teaching clients self-care

5. Select data gathered from visits by a physician or other members of the health team.

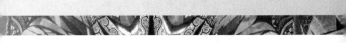

B. SOAP FORMAT

SOAP is an acronym for *s*ubjective data, *o*bjective data, *a*ssessment, and *p*lanning. The SOAP format originated with the problem-oriented medical record but is used increasingly in many different types of records. The acronyms SOAPIE and SOAPIER refer to formats that also include *i*mplementation, *e*valuation, and *r*evision. Many agencies use only the SOAP format. A more recent format is the APIE (*a*ssessment, *p*lan, *i*mplementation, and *e*valuation), which condenses the client data into fewer statements. In APIE, the assessment combines the nursing diagnosis; the plan combines the nursing actions with the expected outcomes; and the implementation and evaluation are the same. Figure 4–1 has examples of a nurse's progress notes using the SOAP, SOAPIER, and APIE formats.

Nursing Progress Notes

SOAP Format

6/6/07	#5	Generalized pruritus
1400	S—	"My skin is itchy on my back and arms, and it's been like this for a week."
	O—	Skin appears clear—no rash or irritation noted. Marks where client has scratched noted on left and right forearms. Allergic to Elastoplast but has not been in contact. No previous history of pruritus.
	A—	Altered comfort (pruritus): cause unknown.

SOAPIER Format

6/6/07	#5	Generalized pruritus
1400	S—	"My skin is itchy on my back and arms, and it's been like this for a week."
	O—	Skin appears clear—no rash or irritation noted. Marks where client has scratched noted on left and right forearms. Allergic to Elastoplast but has not been in contact. No previous history of pruritus.
	A—	Altered comfort (pruritus): cause unknown.
	P—	Instruct not to scratch skin.
	—	Apply calamine lotion as necessary.
	—	Cut nails to avoid scratches.

APIE Format

6/6/07	A—	Generalized pruritus r/t unknown cause
1400		States, "My skin is itchy on my back and arms, and it's been like this for a week." Skin appears clear. No rash or irritations noted. Marks where client has scratched noted on left and right forearms. Allergic to Elastoplast but has not been in contact. No previous history of pruritus.
	P—	Instruct not to scratch skin.
	—	Apply calamine lotion as necessary.
	—	Cut nails to avoid scratches.

P—
— Instructed not to scratch skin.
— Applied calamine lotion to back and arms at 1430 h.
— Cut fingernails to avoid scratches.
— Assess further to determine whether recurrence associated with specific drugs or foods.
— Refer to physician and pharmacist for assessment. —*T. Ritchie, RN*

— Assess further to determine whether recurrence associated with specific drugs or foods.
— Refer to physician and pharmacist for assessment.
I— Instructed not to scratch skin.
   Applied calamine lotion to back and arms at 1430 h.
   Assisted to cut fingernails.
   Notified physician and pharmacist of problem.
E— States, "I'm still itchy. That lotion didn't help."
1600
R— Remove calamine lotion and apply hydrocortisone cream as ordered. —*T. Ritchie, RN*

— Assess further to determine whether recurrence associated with specific drugs or foods.
— Refer to physician and pharmacist for assessment.
I— Instructed not to scratch skin.
   Applied calamine lotion to back and arms at 1430 h.
   Assisted to cut fingernails.
   Notified physician and pharmacist of problem.
E— States, "I'm still itchy. That lotion didn't help." —*T. Ritchie, RN*

Figure 4–1 ■ Examples of nursing progress notes using SOAP, SOAPIER, and APIE formats.

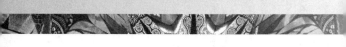

C. EVALUATION

Evaluation is the final phase of the nursing process, in which the nurse determines the client's progress toward goal/outcome achievement and the effectiveness of the nursing care plan:

- Evaluating is determining whether or to what degree client goals have been met.
- Evaluating may be ongoing, intermittent, or terminal.
- Evaluating is purposeful and organized.
- Evaluating uses desired outcomes formulated in the planning phase as criteria for evaluating client progress.

When determining whether a goal has been achieved, the nurse can draw one of three possible conclusions:

1. The goal was met; that is, the client response is the same as the desired outcome.
2. The goal was partially met; that is, either a short-term goal was achieved but the long-term goal was not, or the desired outcome was only partially attained.
3. The goal was not met.

When goals have been partially met or when goals have not been met, two conclusions may be drawn:

1. The care plan may need to be revised because the problem is only partially resolved. The revisions may need to occur during assessing, diagnosing, or planning phases, as well as implementing.

2. The care plan does not need revision because the client merely needs more time to achieve the previously established goal(s). To make this decision, the nurse must assess why the goals are being only partially achieved, including whether the evaluation was conducted too soon.

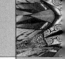

UNIT 5

QUICK REFERENCE

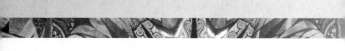

A. STANDARD PRECAUTIONS AND INFECTION CONTROL STRATEGIES

Recommended Infection Control Precautions in Hospitals

Standard Precautions

These precautions are used in the care of all clients regardless of their diagnosis or possible infection status:

- Designed for all clients in hospital
- Apply to (a) blood; (b) all body fluids, excretions, and secretions except sweat; (c) nonintact (broken) skin; and (d) mucous membranes
- Designed to reduce risk of transmission of microorganisms from recognized and unrecognized sources

  1. Cleanse hands after contact with blood, body fluids, secretions, excretions, and contaminated objects regardless if gloves are worn.

     a. Cleanse hands immediately after removing gloves.

     b. Use a nonantimicrobial soap or alcohol-based gel for routine hand cleansing.

     c. Use an antimicrobial agent or an antiseptic agent for the control of specific outbreaks of infection.

  2. Wear clean gloves when touching blood, body fluids, secretions, excretions, and contaminated items (e.g., soiled gowns).

     a. Clean gloves can be unsterile unless they are intended to prevent the entrance of microorganisms into the body.

b. Remove gloves before touching noncontaminated items and surfaces.

c. Cleanse hands immediately after removing gloves.

3. Wear a mask, eye protection, or a face shield if splashes or sprays of blood, body fluids, secretions, or excretions can be expected.

4. Wear a clean, nonsterile gown if client care is likely to result in splashes or sprays of blood, body fluids, secretions, or excretions. The gown is intended to protect clothing.

   a. Remove a soiled gown carefully to avoid the transfer of microorganisms to others (e.g., clients or other health care workers).

   b. Cleanse hands after removing gown.

5. Handle client care equipment that is soiled with blood, body fluids, secretions, or excretions carefully to prevent the transfer of microorganisms to others and to the environment.

   a. Make sure reusable equipment is cleaned and reprocessed correctly.

   b. Dispose of single-use equipment correctly.

6. Handle, transport, and process linen that is soiled with blood, body fluids, secretions, or excretions in a manner to prevent contamination of clothing and the transfer of microorganisms to others and to the environment.

7. Prevent injuries from used equipment such as scalpels or needles, and place them in puncture-resistant containers.

Transmission-Based Precautions

These precautions are used in addition to standard precautions for clients with known or suspected infection that is spread in one of three ways: by airborne or droplet transmission or by contact. The three types of transmission-based precautions may be used alone or in combination, but always *in addition to* standard precautions.

Airborne Precautions

Use standard precautions as well as the following:

1. Place client in a private room that has negative air pressure, 6 to 12 air changes per hour, and discharge of air to the outside or a filtration system for the room air.

2. If a private room is not available, place client with another client who is infected with the same microorganism.

3. Wear a respiratory device (N95 respirator) when entering the room of a client who is known to have or suspected of having primary tuberculosis.

4. Susceptible people should not enter the room of a client who has rubella (measles) or varicella (chickenpox). If they must enter, they should wear a respirator.

5. Limit movement of client outside the room to essential purposes. Place a surgical mask on the client if possible.

Droplet Precautions

Use standard precautions as well as the following:

1. Place client in a private room.

2. If a private room is not available, place client with another client who is infected with the same microorganism.

3. Wear a mask if working within 3 feet of the client.

4. Transport client outside of the room only when necessary and place a surgical mask on the client if possible.

Contact Precautions

Use standard precautions as well as the following:

1. Place client in a private room.

2. If a private room is not available, place client with another client who is infected with the same microorganism.

3. Wear gloves as described in standard precautions.

a. Change gloves after contact with infectious material.

b. Remove gloves before leaving client's room.

c. Cleanse hands immediately after removing gloves. Use an antimicrobial agent.

d. After hand cleansing, do not touch possibly contaminated surfaces or items in the room.

4. Wear a gown (see Standard Precautions) when entering a room if there is a possibility of contact with infected surfaces or items or if the client is incontinent, has diarrhea, has a colostomy, or has wound drainage not contained by a dressing.

a. Remove gown in the client's room.

b. Make sure uniform does not contact possible contaminated surfaces.

5. Limit movement of client outside the room.

6. Dedicate the use of noncritical client care equipment to a single client or to clients with the same infecting microorganisms.

References

Garner, J. S., & the Hospital Infection Control Practices Advisory Committee (HICPAC). (1996). Guidelines for isolation precautions in hospitals. *Infection Control Hospital Epidemiology, 17,* 53–80; and *American Journal of Infection Control, 24,* 24–52.

Bloodborne Pathogens

Sometimes, despite the best practices, the nurse may be exposed to body substances likely to transmit bloodborne pathogens—those microorganisms carried in blood and body fluids that are capable of infecting other persons with serious and difficult-to-treat viral infections, namely hepatitis B virus, hepatitis C virus, and human immunodeficiency virus (HIV). Currently, all health care workers should be vaccinated against hepatitis B, but no vaccines are available for prevention of hepatitis C or HIV. The three major modes of transmission of infectious materials in the clinical setting are the following:

1. Puncture wounds from contaminated needles or other sharps
2. Skin contact, which allows infectious fluids to enter through wounds and broken or damaged skin
3. Mucous membrane contact, which allows infectious fluids to enter through mucous membranes of the eyes, mouth, and nose

It is critical that the nurse follow the next steps to ensure prompt evaluation and treatment, if indicated:

Steps to Follow after Exposure to Bloodborne Pathogens

- Report the incident immediately to appropriate personnel within the agency.
- Complete an injury report.
- Seek appropriate evaluation and follow-up. This includes the following:
  - Identification and documentation of the source individual when feasible and legal
  - Testing of the source for hepatitis B, hepatitis C, and HIV when feasible and consent is given
  - Making results of the test available to the source individual's health care provider
  - Testing of blood of exposed nurse (with consent) for hepatitis B, hepatitis C, and HIV antibodies
  - Postexposure prophylaxis if medically indicated
  - Medical and psychological counseling regarding personal risk of infection or risk of infecting others
- For a puncture/laceration
  - Wash/clean the area with soap and water
  - Initiate first aid and seek treatment if indicated
- For a mucous membrane exposure (eyes, nose, mouth), perform saline or water flush for 5 to 10 minutes.

Postexposure Prophylaxis
Human Immunodeficiency Virus

- For high-risk exposure (high blood volume *and* source with a high HIV titer): three-drug treatment is recommended. Should be started within 1 hour.

- For increased-risk exposure (high blood volume *or* source with a high HIV titer): three-drug treatment is recommended. Should be started within 1 hour.

- For low-risk exposure (*neither* high blood volume *nor* source with a high HIV titer): two-drug treatment is considered. Should be started within 1 hour.

- Drug prophylaxis is for 4 weeks.

- Drug regimens vary. Drugs commonly used are zidovudine, lamivudine, didanosine, and indinavir.

- HIV antibody tests done shortly after exposure (baseline), and 6 weeks, 3 months, and 6 months afterward.

Hepatitis B

- Testing for antibodies to hepatitis B surface antigen (anti-HBs), administering booster dose if not immune

Hepatitis C

- Testing for antibodies to hepatitis C surface antigen (Anti-HCV) and for alanine aminotransferase (ALT) at baseline and 4 to 6 months after exposure

Infection Control Strategies

- Use strict aseptic technique when performing any invasive procedure (e.g., inserting an intravenous needle or catheter, suctioning an airway, and inserting a urinary catheter) and when changing surgical dressings.

- Handle needles and syringes carefully to avoid needle stick injuries.

- Change intravenous tubing and solution containers according to hospital policy (e.g., every 48 to 72 hours).

- Check all sterile supplies for expiration date and intact packaging.

- Prevent urinary infections by maintaining a closed urinary drainage system with a downhill flow of urine; do not irrigate a catheter unless ordered to do so; provide regular catheter care; and keep the drainage bag and spout off the floor.
- Implement measures to prevent impaired skin integrity and to prevent accumulation of secretions in the lungs (e.g., encourage the client to move, cough, and breathe deeply at least every 2 hours).

Preventing Infections in the Home

The nurse teaches the client and family members to do the following:

- Wash hands before handling foods, before eating, after toileting, before and after any required home care treatment, and after touching any body substances (e.g., wound drainage).
- Keep fingernails short, clean, and well-manicured to eliminate rough edges or hangnails, which can harbor microorganisms.
- Do not share personal care items: toothbrush, washcloths, and towels.
- Wash raw fruits and vegetables before eating them.
- Refrigerate all opened and nonpackaged foods.
- Clean used equipment (e.g., emesis basin) with soap and water, and disinfect with a chlorine bleach solution.
- Place contaminated dressings and other disposable items containing body fluids in moisture-proof plastic bags.
- Put used needles in a puncture-resistant container with a screw-top lid. Label so as not to discard in the garbage.
- Clean obviously soiled linen separately from other laundry. Rinse in cold water, wash in hot water if possible, and add a cup of bleach or Lysol to the wash.
- Avoid coughing, sneezing, or breathing directly on others. Cover the mouth and nose to prevent the transmission of airborne microorganisms.

- Be aware of any signs or symptoms of an infection, and report these immediately to the health care provider.
- Maintain a sufficient fluid intake to promote urine production and output. This helps flush the bladder and urethra of microorganisms.

B. COMMON ABBREVIATIONS AND "DO NOT USE" ABBREVIATIONS

Common Abbreviations

Abbreviation	Term
abd	abdomen
ABO	the main blood group system
ac	before meals (ante cibum)
ADL	activities of daily living
ad lib	as desired (ad libitum)
adm	admitted or admission
AM	morning (ante meridiem)
amb	ambulatory
amt	amount
approx	approximately (about)
bid	twice daily (bis in die)
BM (bm)	bowel movement
BP	blood pressure
BR	bed rest
BRP	bathroom privileges
$\bar{c}$	with
C	Celsius (centigrade)
CBC	complete blood count
c/o	complains of
DAT	diet as tolerated
DNR	do not resuscitate
drsg	dressing
Dx	diagnosis
ECG (EKG)	electrocardiogram
F	Fahrenheit
fld	fluid
GI	gastrointestinal

Abbreviation	Term
gtt	drops (guttae)
h (hr)	hour (hora)
H_2O	water
hs	at bedtime (hora somni)
I & O	intake and output
IV	intravenous
LMP	last menstrual period
Lt (lt, L)	left
meds	medications
mL (ml)	milliliter
mod	moderate
neg	negative
Ø	none
#	number
NPO (NBM)	nothing by mouth (nil per os)
NS (N/S)	normal saline
O_2	oxygen
OD	right eye (oculus dexter); overdose
OOB	out of bed
OS	left eye (oculus sinister)
pc	after meals (post cibum)
PE (PX)	physical examination
per	by or through
PM	afternoon (post meridiem)
po	by mouth (per os)
postop	postoperative(ly)
preop	preoperative(ly)
prep	preparation
prn	when necessary (pro re nata)
qid	four times a day (quater in die)
Rt (rt, R)	right
$\bar{s}$	without (sine)
stat	at once, immediately (statim)
tid	three times a day (ter in die)
TO	telephone order
TPR	temperature, pulse, respirations
VO	verbal order
VS (vs)	vital signs
WNL	within normal limits
wt	weight

(continued)

"Do Not Use" List

Abbreviation	Potential Problem	Preferred Term
The minimum required list required by the Joint Commission on Accreditation of Healthcare Organizations		
U (for "unit")	Mistaken as zero, four, or "cc"	Write "unit"
IU (for "international unit")	Mistaken as "IV" (intravenous) or "10" (ten)	Write "international unit"
Q.D., Q.O.D (Latin abbreviation for "once daily" and "every other day")	Mistaken for each other. Period after the "Q" mistaken for an "I" and the "O" mistaken for "I"	Write "daily" and "every other day"
Trailing zero (X.0 mg) (Note: prohibited only for medication-related notations); lack of leading zero (.X mg)	Decimal point is missed	Never write a zero by itself after a decimal point (X mg), and always use a zero before a decimal point (0.X mg)
MS, MSO₄, and MgSO₄	Confused for one another. Can mean "morphine sulfate" or "magnesium sulfate"	Write "morphine sulfate" or "magnesium sulfate"
In addition to the "minimum required list" above, the following should be considered when expanding the "do not use" list:		
μg (for "microgram")	Mistaken for "mg" (milligrams), resulting in 1000-fold overdose	Write "mcg"
H.S. (for "half-strength" or Latin abbreviation for "bedtime")	Mistaken for either "half-strength" or "hour of sleep" ("at bedtime"). "q.H.S." mistaken for "every hour." All can result in a dosing error	Write out "half-strength" or "at bedtime"
T.I.W. (for "three times a week")	Mistaken for "three times a day" or "twice weekly" resulting in an overdose	Write "3 times weekly" or "three times weekly"
S.C. or S.Q. (for "subcutaneous")	Mistaken as "SL" (for "sublingual") and as "5 every"	Write "Sub-Q," "subQ," or "subcutaneously"

Abbreviation	Potential Problem	Preferred Term
D/C (for "discharge")	Interpreted as "discontinue whatever medications follow" (typically discharge medications)	Write "discharge"
c.c.	Mistaken for "U" (units) when poorly written	Write "ml" or "milliliters"
A.S., A.D., A.U. (Latin abbreviation for "left ear," "right ear," and "both ears," respectively)	Mistaken for "OS," "OD," and "OU," etc.	Write "left ear," "right ear," or "both ears"

Note: From "2006 National Patient Safety Goals—FAQs," by Joint Commission on Accreditation of Healthcare Organizations, 2006. Retrieved April 30, 2006, from http://www.jointcommission.org/NR/rdonlyres/2329F8F5-6EC5-4E21-B932-54B2B7D53F00/0/06_dnu_list.pdf

C. MEDICAL TERMINOLOGY: ROOT WORDS, PREFIXES, AND SUFFIXES

Word Element	Meaning
Root Words	
Circulatory System	
cardio	heart
angio, vaso	vessel
hem, hema, hemato	blood
vena, phlebo	vein
arteria	artery
lympho	lymph
thrombo	clot (of blood)
embolus	moving clot
Digestive System	
bucca	cheek
os, stomato	mouth
gingiva	gum
glossa	tongue
pharyngo	pharynx
esophago	esophagus
gastro	stomach
hepato	liver
cholecyst	gallbladder
pancreas	pancreas
entero	intestines
duodeno	duodenum
jejuno	jejunum
ileo	ileum
caeco	cecum
appendeco	appendix
colo	colon
recto	rectum
ano, procto	anus

Word Element	Meaning
Skeletal System	
skeleto	skeleton
Respiratory System	
naso, rhino	nose
tonsillo	tonsil
laryngo	larynx
tracheo	trachea
bronchus, broncho	bronchus (pl. bronchi)
pulmo, pneuma, pneum	lung (sac with air)
Nervous System	
neuro	nerve
cerebrum	brain
oculo, ophthalmo	eye
oto	ear
psych, psycho	mind
Urinary System	
urethro	urethra
cysto	bladder
uretero	ureter
reni, reno, nephro	kidney
pyleo	pelvis of kidney
uro	urine
Female Reproductive System	
vulvo	vulva
perineo	perineum
labio	labium (pl. labia)
vagino, colpo	vagina
cervico	cervix
utero	womb; uterus
tubo, salpingo	fallopian tube
ovario, oophoro	ovary
Male Reproductive System	
orchido	testes
Regions of the Body	
crani, cephalo	head
cervico, tracheo	neck
thoraco	chest
abdomino	abdomen
dorsum	back
Tissues	
cutis, dermato	skin
lipo	fat

C. Medical Terminology (continued)

Word Element	Meaning
musculo, myo	muscle
osteo	bone
myelo	marrow
chondro	cartilage
Miscellaneous	
cyto	cell
genetic	formation, origin
gram	tracing or mark
graph	writing, description
kinesis	motion
meter	measure
oligo	small, few
phobia	fear
photo	light
pyo	pus
scope	instrument for visual examination
roentgen	x-ray
lapar	flank; through the abdominal wall

Prefixes

a, an, ar	without or not
ab	away from
acro	extremities
ad	toward, to
adeno	glandular
aero	air
ambi	around, on both sides
amyl	starch
ante	before, forward
anti	against, counteracting
bi	double
bili	bile
bio	life
bis	two
brachio	arm
brady	slow
broncho	bronchus (pl. bronchi)
cardio	heart
cervico	neck
chole	gall or bile
cholecysto	gallbladder

Word Element	Meaning
circum	around
co	together
contra	against, opposite
costo	ribs
cyto	cell
cysto	bladder
demi	half
derma	skin
dis	from
dorso	back
dys	abnormal, difficult
electro	electric
en	into, in, within
encephal	brain
entero	intestine
equi	equal
eryth	red
ex	out, out of, away from
extra	outside of, in addition to
ferro	iron
fibro	fiber
fore	before, in front of
gastro	stomach
glosso	tongue
glyco	sugar
hemi	half
hemo	blood
hepa, hepato	liver
histo	tissue
homo	same
hydro	water
hygro	moisture
hyper	too much, high
hypo	under, decreased
hyster	uterus
ileo	ileum
in	in, within, into
inter	between
intra	within
intro	in, within, into
juxta	near, close to
laryngo	larynx

C. Medical Terminology *(continued)*

Word Element	Meaning
latero	side
lapar	abdomen
leuk	white
macro	large, big
mal	bad, poor
mast	breast
medio	middle
mega, megalo	large, great
meno	menses
mono	single
multi	many
myelo	bone marrow, spinal cord
myo	muscle
neo	new
nephro	kidney
neuro	nerve
nitro	nitrogen
noct	night
non	not
ob	against, in front of
oculo	eye
odonto	tooth
ophthalmo	eye
ortho	straight, normal
os	mouth, bone
osteo	bone
oto	ear
pan	all
para	beside, accessory to
path	disease
ped	child, foot
per	by, through
peri	around
pharyngo	pharynx
phlebo	vein
photo	light
phren	diaphragm, mind
pneumo	air, lungs
pod	foot
poly	many, much

Word Element	Meaning
post	after
pre	before
proct	rectum
pseudo	false
psych	mind
pyel	pelvis of the kidney
pyo	pus
pyro	fever, heat
quadri	four
radio	radiation
re	back, again
reno	kidney
retro	backward
rhin	nose
sacro	sacrum
salpingo	fallopian tube
sarco	flesh
sclero	hard, hardening
semi	half
sex	six
skeleto	skeleton
steno	narrowing, constriction
sub	under
super	above, excess
supra	above
syn	together
tachy	fast
thyro	thyroid, gland
trache	trachea
trans	across, over
tri	three
ultra	beyond
un	not, back, reversal
uni	one
uretero	ureter
urethro	urethra
uro	urine, urinary organs
vaso	vessel

Suffixes

able	able to
algia	pain

C. Medical Terminology *(continued)*

Word Element	Meaning
cele	tumor, swelling
centesis	surgical puncture to remove fluid
cide	killing, destructive
cule	little
cyte	cell
ectasia	dilating, stretching
ectomy	excision, surgical removal of
emia	blood
esis	action
form	shaped like
genesis, genetic	formation, origin
gram	tracing, mark
graph	writing
ism	condition
itis	inflammation
ize	to treat
lith	stone, calculus
lithiasis	presence of stones
lysis	disintegration
megaly	enlargement
meter	instrument that measures
oid	likeness, resemblance
oma	tumor
opathy	disease of
orrhaphy	surgical repair
osis	disease, condition of
ostomy	to form an opening or outlet
otomy	to incise
pexy	fixation
phage	ingesting
phobia	fear
plasty	plastic surgery
plegia	paralysis
rhage	to burst forth
rhea	excessive discharge
rhexis	rupture
scope	lighted instrument for visual examination
scopy	to examine visually
stomy	to form an opening
tomy	incision into
uria	urine

D. WEIGHT AND VOLUME CONVERSIONS AND EQUIVALENTS

Prefix	Abbreviations	Numerical	Value
Basic Metric Units			
kilo	k	1000	one thousand
hecto	h	100	one hundred
deka	dk	10	ten
deci	d	0.1	one-tenth
centi	c	0.01	one-hundredth
milli	M	0.001	one-thousandth
micro	mc, μ	0.000001	one-millionth

Metric Weight Equivalents

1 kg (kilogram)	= 1000 g (grams)
1 g (gram)	= 1000 mg (milligrams)
1 mg (milligram)	= 1000 mcg, μg (micrograms)

Approximate Weight Equivalents: Metric and Apothecaries' Systems

Metric	Apothecaries'
0.1 mg	1/600 grain (gr)
0.6 mg	1/100 grain
1 mg	1/60 grain
4 mg	1/15 grain
6 mg	1/10 grain
10 mg	1/6 grain
15 mg	1/4 grain
30 mg	1/2 grain
60 mg	1 grain
500 mg (0.5 g)	7 1/2 grains
600 mg (0.6 g)	10 grains
1 g (1000 mg)	15 grains
2 g	30 grains
4 g	60 grains (1 dram)

D. Weight and Volume Conversions and Equivalents *(continued)*

Metric	Apothecaries'
7.5 g	120 grains (2 drams)
30 g	1 ounce (8 drams)
1000 g	2.2 pounds (1 kilogram)

Approximate Volume Equivalents: Metric, Apothecaries', and Household Systems

Metric	Apothecaries'	Household
0.06 mL	1 minim (m)	1 drop (gt)
0.3 mL	5 minims	5 drops (gtt)
0.6 mL	10 minims	10 drops (gtt)
1 mL (1 cubic cm)	15 minims	15 drops (gtt)
2 mL	30 minims	30 drops (gtt)
3 mL	45 minims	45 drops (gtt)
4 mL	60 minims (1 fluid dram [ℨ])	60 drops (1 teaspoon [tsp])
8 mL	2 fluid drams	2 teaspoons
15 mL	4 fluid drams	4 teaspoons (1 tablespoon)
30 mL	8 fluid drams (1 fluid ounce [ℨ])	2 tablespoons
60 mL	2 fluid ounces	
90 mL	3 fluid ounces	
200 mL	6 fluid ounces	1 teacup
250 mL	8 fluid ounces	1 large glass
500 mL	16 fluid ounces (1 pint [pt])	1 pint
1000 mL (1 liter)	2 pints (1 quart [qt])	1 quart
4000 mL 1 gallon (gal)	4 quarts	

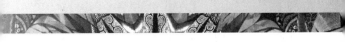

E. LABORATORY VALUES

The ranges for normal values may vary from laboratory to laboratory; therefore, always check with each agency for its own normal range and for the particular testing method, and, if indicated, for the population for which the set of values is described. All values should be interpreted within the context of the client's health status. Refer to Chapter 52 of *Fundamentals of Nursing* for a thorough discussion of fluids, electrolytes, and acid–base balance.

Table A: Complete Blood Count with Clinical Implications

Component	Normal Findings (Adult)	Possible Causes of Abnormal Findings	
		Increased	Decreased
Red blood cell count (RBC) The number of RBCs per cubic millimeter (mm^3).	Male: 4.5–5.3 million/ mm^3 Female: 4.1–5.1 million/ mm^3	Primary polycythemia (e.g., polycythemia vera) Secondary polycythemia or erythrocytosis—usually caused by oxygen need (e.g., chronic lung disease, congenital heart defects)	Abnormal loss of erythrocytes Abnormal destruction of erythrocytes Lack of needed elements or hormones for erythrocyte production Bone marrow suppression
Hemoglobin (Hgb) Composed of a pigment (heme), which contains iron, and a protein (globin).	Male: 13.8–18 g/dL Female: 12–16 g/dL	Polycythemia	Blood loss Hemolytic anemia Bone marrow suppression Sickle cell anemia

Hematocrit (Hct)

The hematocrit or packed cell volume (Hct, PCV, or crit) is a fast way to determine the percentage of RBCs in the plasma. The Hct is reported as a percentage because it is the proportion of RBCs to the plasma.

Male: 37–49%
Female: 36–46%

Polycythemia
Dehydration
Burns

Blood loss
Overhydration
Dietary deficiency
Anemia

Red blood cell indices (RBC indices)

Mean corpuscular volume (MCV): the mean or average size of the individual RBC.

Male: 78–100 mm^3
Female: 78–102 mm^3

Liver disease
Alcoholism
Pernicious anemia

Iron deficiency anemia
Lead poisoning

Mean corpuscular hemoglobin (MCH): amount of Hgb present in one cell.

25–35 pg

Rarely seen

Iron deficiency anemia

Mean corpuscular hemoglobin concentration (MCHC): the proportion of each cell occupied by Hgb.

31–37%

Rarely seen

Iron deficiency anemia

(continued)

E. Laboratory Values   163

Table A: Complete Blood Count with Clinical Implications *(continued)*

Component	Normal Findings (Adult)	Possible Causes of Abnormal Findings	
		Increased	Decreased
White blood cell count (WBC) Count of the total number of WBCs in a cubic millimeter of blood.	4,500–11,000/mm^3	Leukocytosis Infection	Leukopenia Autoimmune disease
Differential count The proportion of each of the five types of WBCs in a sample of 100 WBCs.			
Neutrophils	55–70%	Stress Acute infection	Viral diseases Some drugs (e.g., chemotherapy, antibiotics such as nafcillin, penicillin, and cephalosporins) Radiation therapy
Lymphocytes	20–40%	Viral infection Mononucleosis	Adrenal corticosteroids and other immunosuppressive drugs

		Increased	Decreased
Monocytes	2–8%	Tuberculosis Chronic bacterial infections Lymphocytic leukemia Chronic inflammatory disorders Tuberculosis Protozoan infections (e.g., malaria, Rocky Mountain spotted fever) Chronic ulcerative colitis	Autoimmune diseases (e.g., lupus erythematosus) Severe malnutrition Drug therapy: prednisone
Eosinophils	1–4%	Allergic reactions (e.g., asthma, hay fever, or hypersensitivity to a drug) Parasitic infestations (e.g., roundworms)	Corticosteroid therapy
Basophils	0–2%	Leukemia	Acute allergic reaction Corticosteroids Acute infections

(continued)

Table A: Complete Blood Count with Clinical Implications *(continued)*

Component	Normal Findings (Adult)	Possible Causes of Abnormal Findings	
		Increased	Decreased
Platelet count			
Platelets are fragments of cyto-plasm that function in blood coagulation.	150,000–350,000/mm^3	Malignant tumors Polycythemia vera	Idiopathic (unknown cause) Thrombocytopenic purpura Viral infections Acquired immunodeficiency syndrome Systemic lupus erythematosus Chemotherapy drugs Some types of anemias

Note: Reprinted with permission from Corbett, J.V. (2004). *Laboratory tests and diagnostic procedures with nursing diagnoses* (6th ed.). Upper Saddle River, NJ: Pearson Prentice Hall.

Table B: Common Blood Chemistry Tests with Clinical Implications

Test	Normal Findings (Adult)	Significance	Possible Causes of Increased	Possible Causes of Decreased
Liver Function Tests				
Alanine aminotransferase (ALT), formerly known as serum pyretic transaminase (SGPT)	Men: 10–55 U/L Women: 7–30 U/L	Marker of hepatic injury; more specific of liver damage than AST.	Hepatitis; infectious mononucleosis; acute pancreatitis; acute myocardial infarction (MI); heart failure.	Not clinically significant.
Aspartate aminotransferase (AST), formerly known as serum glutamic-oxaloacetic transaminase (SGOT)	Men: 10–40 U/L Women: 9–25 U/L	Found in heart, liver, and skeletal muscle. Can also be used to indicate liver injury.	Liver diseases (e.g., hepatitis, alcoholism, drug toxicity); acute MI; anemias; skeletal muscle diseases.	Chronic renal dialysis; vitamin B_6 deficiency.
Albumin	Adults: 3.5–4.8 g/dL or 35–48 g/L Panic value: <1.5 g/dL	Is a protein produced by the liver.	No pathology causes the liver to produce more albumin. An increased level reflects dehydration.	Chronic liver dysfunction; acquired immunodeficiency syndrome; severe burns; malnutrition; renal disease; acute and chronic infections.

(continued)

Table B: Common Blood Chemistry Tests with Clinical Implications *(continued)*

Test	Normal Findings (Adult)	Significance	Possible Causes of Increased	Possible Causes of Decreased
Alkaline phosphatase	Adults: 25–100 U/L	Found in the tissues of the liver, bone, intestine, kidney, and placenta. Used as an index of liver and bone disease when correlated with other clinical findings.	Liver disease; bone disease; hyperparathyroidism; MI; chronic renal failure; heart failure.	Malnutrition; pernicious anemia and severe anemias; hypothyroidism; magnesium and zinc deficiency (nutritional).
Ammonia	Adults: 35–65 mg/dL	The liver converts ammonia, a byproduct of protein metabolism, into urea, which is excreted by the kidneys.	Liver disease; cirrhosis; Reye's syndrome; gastrointestinal hemorrhage.	Renal failure.

Bilirubin	Adults: Total: 0.3–1.0 mg/dL Direct: 0.0–0.2 mg/dL Indirect: 0.1–1.0 mg/dL Panic value: >12 mg/dL	Results from the breakdown of hemoglobin in the red blood cells; removed from the body by the liver, which excretes it into the bile.	Total: hepatitis; obstruction of the common bile or hepatic ducts; pernicious anemia; sickle cell anemia. Direct: cancer of the head of the pancreas; choledocholithiasis. Indirect: hemolytic anemias; drug toxicity; transfusion reaction.	Not clinically significant.
Gamma-glutamyl transferase (GGT)	Men: 1–94 U/L Women: 1–70 U/L	Found primarily in the liver, kidney, prostate, and spleen. Is more specific for the hepatobiliary system.	Liver disease; alcohol abuse.	Not clinically significant.
Prothrombin	11–13 seconds Critical value: >20 seconds for nonanticoagulated persons	A protein produced by the liver for clotting of blood.	Liver disease, damage; vitamin K deficiency; obstruction of common bile duct; deficiency of factors II, V, VII, or X.	Thrombophlebitis; malignant tumor.

(continued)

Table B: Common Blood Chemistry Tests with Clinical Implications *(continued)*

Test	Normal Findings (Adult)	Significance	Possible Causes of Increased	Possible Causes of Decreased
Cardiac Markers				
Creatine kinase (CK)	Total: Men: 38–174 U/L Women: 26–140 U/L Isoenzymes: MM (CK_3): 96–100% MB (CK_2): 0–6% BB (CK_1): 0%	An enzyme found in the heart and skeletal muscles. Has three isoenzymes: BB (CK_1), MB (CK_2), and MM (CK_3).	Total: acute MI; myocarditis; after open heart surgery; acute cerebrovascular dystrophy; chronic alcoholism. CK isoenzymes: MB (CK_2): Myocardial infarct; myocardial ischemia; angina pectoris.	Not clinically significant.
Myoglobin	5–70 ng/mL	After an MI, serum levels of myoglobin rise in 2–4 hours, making it an early marker for muscle damage in MI.	MI; angina; other muscle injury (e.g., trauma); renal failure; rhabdomyolysis.	Rheumatoid arthritis; myasthenia gravis.

Troponin I	Troponin I: <0.35 ng/mL	Cardiac troponin is highly concentrated in the heart muscle. This test is used in the early diagnosis of MI. After an MI, troponin I begins to increase in 4–6 hours and remains elevated for 5–7 days. Troponin T begins to increase in 3–4 hours and remains elevated for 10–14 days.	Troponin I: small infarct; myocardial injury.
Troponin T	Critical value: >1.5 ng/mL Troponin T: <0.2 ng/mL		Troponin T: acute MI; unstable angina; myocarditis.
			Not clinically significant.

(continued)

Table B: Common Blood Chemistry Tests with Clinical Implications *(continued)*

Test	Normal Findings (Adult)	Significance	Possible Causes of Increased	Possible Causes of Decreased
Brain natriuretic peptide (BNP)	<100 pg/mL or <100 ng/L	A hormone produced by the ventricles of the heart and is a marker of ventricular systolic and diastolic dysfunction. This test is useful in diagnosing and guiding treatment of heart failure.	Heart failure; symptomatic cardiac volume overload; paroxysmal atrial tachycardia.	Not clinically significant.
Lipoprotein Profile				
Cholesterol	Adults, desirable: <200 mg/dL	This test is an important screening test for heart disease.	Type II familial hypercholesterolemia; biliary cirrhosis; chronic renal failure; poorly controlled diabetes mellitus; alcoholism; diet high in cholesterol and fats.	Severe hepatocellular disease; hyperthyroidism; malnutrition; chronic anemias; severe burns.

Test	Reference Value	Description	Increased	Decreased
High-density lipoprotein cholesterol (HDL-C)	Men: 35–65 mg/dL Women: 35–80 mg/dL	A class of lipoproteins produced by the liver and intestines. The "good" cholesterol.	HDL excess; chronic liver disease; long-term aerobic or vigorous exercise.	Familial hypolipoproteinemia; hypertriglyceridemia (familial); poorly controlled diabetes mellitus; chronic renal failure.
Low-density lipoprotein (LDL)	Adults, desirable: <130 mg/dL	Up to 70% of the total serum cholesterol is present in the LDL. The "bad" cholesterol.	Familial type 2 hyperlipidemia; secondary causes can include diet high in cholesterol and saturated fat; nephritic syndrome; multiple myeloma; diabetes mellitus; chronic renal failure.	Hypolipoproteinemia; hyperthyroidism; chronic anemias; severe hepatocellular disease.
Triglycerides	Desirable: <150 mg/dL	This test evaluates suspected atherosclerosis and measures the body's ability to metabolize fat.	Hypolipoproteinemia; liver disease; renal disease; hypothyroidism; pancreatitis; MI.	Malnutrition; hyperthyroidism; brain infarction; chronic obstructive lung disease.

Table C: Serum Electrolytes

Test	Normal Findings (Adult)	Possible Causes of Increased	Possible Causes of Decreased
Sodium	135–145 mEq/L	Cushing's syndrome Dehydration Diabetes insipidus Excessive intravenous sodium Insufficient water intake Impaired renal function	Severe burns Addison's disease Diabetic ketoacidosis Diuretic therapy Excessive gastrointestinal tract loss Water intoxication
Potassium	3.5–5.0 mEq/L	Acidosis Diabetic ketoacidosis Hypoaldosteronism Massive crushing tissue destruction Renal failure Use of potassium-sparing diuretics	Alkalosis Cushing's syndrome Diarrhea (severe) Diuretic therapy Gastrointestinal fistula Pyloric obstruction Starvation Vomiting Alcoholism Burns

Chloride	95–105 mEq/L	Cushing's syndrome Dehydration Hypernatremia Metabolic acidosis Respiratory alkalosis Kidney dysfunction	Overhydration Addison's disease Burns (severe) Diarrhea Diuretic use Metabolic alkalosis Chronic respiratory acidosis Vomiting Gastric suctioning
Calcium (total)	4.5–5.5 mEq/L or 8.5–10.5 mg/dL	Total calcium: Hyperparathyroidism Cancers Hyperthyroidism Prolonged immobility Paget's disease	Total calcium: Reduced albumin Hypoparathyroidism Alkalosis Acute pancreatitis Vitamin D deficiency
Calcium (ionized)	56% of total calcium (2.5 mEq/L or 4.0–5.0 mg/dL)	Ionized calcium: Hypoparathyroidism Excess vitamin D intake	Ionized calcium: Acute pancreatitis Diabetic acidosis Hyperventilation Vitamin D deficiency

(continued)

Table C: Serum Electrolytes *(continued)*

Test	Normal Findings (Adult)	Possible Causes of Increased	Possible Causes of Decreased
Magnesium	1.5–2.5 mEq/L or 2.5–4.5 mg/dL	Addison's disease Dehydration Diabetic ketoacidosis Excessive use of magnesium-containing antacids Hypothyroidism Renal disorders	Hemodialysis Blood transfusions Chronic alcoholism Chronic renal disease Hypoparathyroidism Hyperthyroidism Severe burns
Phosphate (phosphorus)	1.8–2.6 mEq/L or 2.5–4.5 mg/dL	Hypocalcemia Hypoparathyroidism Renal disease Skeletal disease Liver disease Bone metastasis	Malabsorption Chronic alcoholism Diabetes mellitus Hypercalcemia Hyperparathyroidism Vitamin D deficiency
Serum osmolality	280–300 mOsm/kg water	Hypernatremia Dehydration Hyperglycemia Chronic renal disease Diabetes insipidus	Malnutrition Hyponatremia Fluid volume excess Syndrome of inappropriate antidiuretic hormone secretion (SIADH)

Table D: Arterial Blood Gases

Test	Normal Findings (Adult)	Possible Causes of Increased	Possible Causes of Decreased
pH	7.35–7.45	Alkalosis (metabolic and respiratory)	Acidosis (metabolic and respiratory)
PaO_2	80–100 mm Hg	Administration of high concentration of oxygen	Chronic lung disease
			Anemia
$PaCO_2$	35–45 mm Hg	Respiratory acidosis or compensated metabolic alkalosis	Respiratory alkalosis or compensated metabolic acidosis
HCO_3	22–26 mEq/L	Metabolic alkalosis	Metabolic acidosis
Base excess	–2 to +2 mEq/L	Metabolic alkalosis	Metabolic acidosis
Oxygen saturation	95–98%	Polycythemia	Anemia
			Cardiac decompensation
			Respiratory disorders

Table E: Urine Chemistry

| Test | Specimen | Normal Values | | Possible Etiologies | |
		Conventional Units	SI Units	Higher	Lower
Bilirubin	Random	Negative	Negative	Cirrhosis; gallstone; hepatic obstruction; hepatitis	—
Calcium	24h	100–300 mg/day	2.5–7.5 mmol/day	Bone metastases; hyperparathyroidism; breast and bladder cancers	Calcium and vitamin D malabsorption; hypoparathyroidism; renal disease
Creatinine Male Female	24h	0.8–1.8 g/day 0.6–1.6 g/day	7.1–17.7 mmol/day 5.3–15.9 mmol/day	Acromegaly; diabetes mellitus; hyperthyroidism	Heart failure; renal disease; shock; hypothyroidism
Creatinine clearance Male Female	24h	70–150 mL/min 85–132 mL/min	1.42–2.25 mL/sec 1.42–2.25 mL/sec	Exercise; pregnancy; high cardiac output syndromes	Impaired kidney function; heart failure; cirrhosis; shock

Glucose	Random	Negative	Negative	Cushing's syndrome; diabetes mellitus; pregnancy
Hemoglobin	Random	Negative	Negative	Hematuria: trauma to kidneys; glomerulonephritis; hemolytic transfusion reaction; urinary tract infections; urinary calculi; hemoglobinuria; burns; transfusion reaction; sickle cell anemia
Ketone bodies	Random dipstick	Negative	Negative	Diabetes (uncontrolled); fasting; high-protein diet; starvation; pregnancy

(continued)

Table E: Urine Chemistry (continued)

| Test | Specimen | Normal Values | | Possible Etiologies | |
		Conventional Units	SI Units	Higher	Lower
pH	Random	4.6–8.0	4.6–8.0	Alkalosis; chronic renal failure; diuretic use; gastric suction; salicylate intoxication; urinary tract infection; vegetable diet; vomiting	Acidosis; dehydration; starvation; urinary tract infections
Protein (dipstick)	Random	Negative	Negative	Congestive heart failure; glomerulosclerosis; lupus erythematosus; multiple myeloma; nephrotic syndrome	—

Specific gravity	Random	1.010–1.025	Albuminuria; dehydration; diarrhea; glycosuria; presence of contrast medium; vomiting	Diabetes insipidus; overhydration; renal disease
Uric acid	24h	250–750 mg/day	1.5–4.5 mmol/day	Gout; hepatic disease; sickle cell anemia	Chronic glomerulonephritis; lead toxicity; nephritis

References

Corbett, J. V. (2004). *Laboratory tests and diagnostic procedures with nursing diagnoses* (6th ed.). Upper Saddle River, NJ: Pearson Prentice Hall.

Fischbach, F. (2004). *A manual of laboratory diagnostic tests* (6th ed.). Philadelphia: Lippincott Williams and Wilkins.

Van Leeuwen, A. M., Krampitz, T. R., & Smith, L. (2006). *Laboratory and diagnostic tests with nursing implications* (2nd ed.). Philadelphia: F. A. Davis.

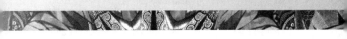

F. COMMON DIAGNOSTIC STUDIES

Test	Purpose
Blood	
Complete blood count (CBC)	To determine hemoglobin (Hgb), hematocrit (Hct), and erythrocyte, or red blood cell (RBC) count and assess the blood's ability to carry oxygen; to determine the leukocyte, or white blood cell (WBC) count, which signals infection when elevated.
Serum electrolytes (Na^+, K^+, Mg^{2+}, Ca^{2+}, H^+)	To determine electrolyte and acid–base imbalances.
Arterial blood gas (ABG) analysis	To determine the adequacy of alveolar gas exchange and evaluate the ability of the lungs and kidneys to maintain the acid–base balance of the body fluids. ABGs include pH, P_{CO_2}, bicarbonate, P_{O_2} and oxygen saturation, and base excess.
Fasting blood sugar (FBS) test	To detect presence of glucose in the blood, which may indicate metabolic disorders (e.g., diabetes mellitus).
Glucose tolerance test (GTT)	To determine ability to tolerate a standard glucose load (insulin response) without spillage over into the urine.
Blood urea nitrogen (BUN) or creatinine	To assess urinary excretion.
Sputum	
Sputum culture and sensitivity test	To determine the presence of pathogenic bacteria and bacterial sensitivity to various antibiotics.
Acid-fast bacilli (AFB) test	To determine the presence of acid-fast bacilli, indicating, for example, active tuberculosis.
Cytologic tests	To determine the presence of abnormal or malignant cells.

(continued)

183

F. Common Diagnostic Studies *(continued)*

Test	Purpose
Urine	
Urinalysis (UA)	To detect urinary tract infections and glucose in the urine.
Urine culture and sensitivity test	To determine the presence of pathogenic bacteria and bacterial sensitivity to various antibiotics.
Stool	
Guaiac test	To determine the presence of occult blood and bleeding in the gastrointestinal tract.
Ova and parasite tests (O & P)	To determine the presence of a parasitic infection of the intestine.
Radiologic	
Chest roentgenogram (CXR)	To identify lung disease and heart size and location.
Upper gastrointestinal (UGI) test	To identify lesions in the esophagus, stomach, and duodenum after barium, a contrast medium, is swallowed.
Lower gastrointestinal (LGI) test	To identify lesions of the large bowel after a barium enema.
Scan of the head, chest, bone, or entire body	A noninvasive x-ray procedure that distinguishes minor differences in the radiodensity of soft tissues (e.g., a tumor in liver tissue).
Other	
Electrocardiogram (ECG or EKG)	To determine the presence of cardiac disease.
Exercise stress test	To determine the client's ability to obtain and maintain maximum heart rate of 85% for predicted age and sex with no cardiac symptoms or ECG (EKG) change.
Tuberculin (TB) skin test	To detect tuberculosis infection; however, does not indicate whether the infection is active or dormant.

G. NURSING INTERVENTIONS FOR ENDOSCOPIC EXAMINATIONS

Examination	Nursing Intervention		
	Preprocedure	During Procedure	Postprocedure
Laryngoscopy or bronchoscopy	Explain the procedure, and clarify the client's concerns. Explain that a local spray or gargle will be given or that medications will be injected through a needle in the vein; that the client will rest the teeth against a small plastic mouthpiece; and that the procedure is painless but some pressure may be felt. Explain that the test will take about 30–60 minutes. Assess vital signs, sputum, and character of respirations for baseline data.	Assist the physician as required, for example, to hold the head-piece or to move the client's head. Monitor the client's pulse and respirations. Support the client using touch and verbal communication.	1. Monitor vital signs q30min or as needed during the recovery period, and compare results to baseline data. 2. Withhold fluids until the gag reflex is restored and the client is conscious. 3. Position the client as ordered or indicated. Place the unconscious client in the lateral position so that secretions are not aspirated. 4. Inspect the client's sputum for blood caused by tissue damage.

(continued)

G. Nursing Interventions for Endoscopic Examinations *(continued)*

Examination	Nursing Intervention		
	Preprocedure	During Procedure	Postprocedure
	Remove dentures, necklaces, earrings, hairpins, and combs. Ensure good oral hygiene. Ensure that client is NPO for 6–8 hours beforehand. Confirm that the client is not allergic to any medications that will be given. Administer analgesic, sedative, antianxiety agent, and medication to dry secretions, if ordered.		5. Observe the client for signs of dyspnea, stridor, and shortness of breath, which may result from laryngeal edema or laryngospasm. 6. Provide ice chips and warm saline gargles or throat lozenges, and administer ordered analgesics as required for throat discomfort. 7. Advise the client to contact the physician should difficulty with breathing, blood in sputum, fever, or pain occur.

Esophagoscopy, gastroscopy, and duodenoscopy	As above for bronchoscopy, with the exception of assessing sputum. Explain that the client may feel pressure in the stomach as the tube is moved about and feel fullness or bloating, like that after eating a large meal.	As above for bronchoscopy. Administer oral simethicone (Mylicon) before test if ordered; it decreases air bubbles in the stomach. If atropine is given intravenously to reduce gastrointestinal spasm, carefully monitor the client's pulse rate. Atropine increases the heart rate.	1. Follow steps 1–3 and 6, as for bronchoscopy. 2. Inspect vomitus for blood, and test it for occult blood if agency practice indicates. 3. Advise the client to contact the physician if client experiences persistent difficulty swallowing, pain, fever, blood in vomitus, or black stools.
Cystoscopy	Assess vital signs, frequency of urination, dysuria, and amount and consistency of urine for baseline data. Administer enema, if ordered. A clear bowel is necessary if x-ray studies are planned. If a general anesthetic is being given, ensure that client is NPO for 6–8 hours beforehand.	Support the client emotionally. Monitor vital signs. Label appropriately any specimens taken. Assist the primary care provider as requested.	1. Monitor vital signs, urination, and urine, and compare with baseline data. 2. Position the unconscious client appropriately (as for bronchoscopy). 3. Inspect the client's urine for blood; report bright red bleeding.

(continued)

G. Nursing Interventions for Endoscopic Examinations *(continued)*

Examination	Nursing Intervention		
	Preprocedure	During Procedure	Postprocedure
	For the client having a local anesthetic, provide appropriate fluid intake, if ordered, to ensure an adequate flow of urine for the collection of specimens. Administer sedative and medication to dry secretions, if ordered.		4. Report inability to urinate by 8 hours. 5. Encourage increased fluid intake to decrease irritation of urinary tissue. 6. If dyes were used in the procedure, warn the client that the urine may be an unusual color. 7. Administer analgesics, as ordered. 8. Advise the client to report persistent difficulty passing urine, bright blood in urine, pain, or fever.
Anoscopy, proctoscopy, sigmoidoscopy, and colonoscopy	Assess vital signs and consistency of feces for baseline data. Ensure appropriate preexamination diet and fluid intake.	Support the client physically in the genupectoral position, as needed. Monitor pulse and respiratory rates.	1. Monitor vital signs and compare with baseline data. 2. Inspect the next few bowel movements for blood.

Administer enemas until returns are clear, or suppository as ordered, the morning of the examination.

Ensure that the client voids before the examination. The pressure during the procedure may injure a full bladder.

Administer sedative beforehand, if ordered.

Just before the endoscope is inserted, explain that the client may experience (a) sensation of having to move bowels (due to the pressure of the instrument) and (b) abdominal cramping when distending bowel with air.

Label appropriately any specimens taken.

Support the client emotionally. Acknowledge feelings the client experiences (e.g., cramps) and ensure the client that they are not unusual.

3. Allow the client to rest. This procedure may be physically and emotionally tiring.
4. Provide fluids and food.

H. Studies of the Gastrointestinal Tract

		Nursing Intervention	
Name	Description	Preprocedure	Postprocedure
Barium swallow	The client swallows barium, and the pharynx and esophagus are outlined on x-ray film.	Procedure lasts 30 minutes. Client is given a chalky substance (liquid barium) to drink.	Encourage fluids and activity to prevent constipation. Observe stool for whitish color indicating client has passed barium in stool. Notify primary care provider if barium does not pass in 2–3 days (a laxative may be required).
Upper gastrointestinal (UGI) series	The client swallows barium, and x-ray films are taken of its course through the esophagus, stomach, and duodenum.	Client must fast 4–6 hours before the examination. The client is given a chalky substance (liquid barium) to drink. Procedure lasts from 30 minutes to 1 hour. Client may experience a feeling of fullness. Client may need to assume several positions on the x-ray table.	Encourage fluids and activity to prevent constipation. Observe stool for whitish color, indicating client has passed barium in stool. Client may require a laxative or enema if client is constipated or does not pass barium in 2–3 days.

| Lower gastrointestinal (LGI) series (barium enema) | A barium enema is given, and x-ray films are taken of the large intestine. | A laxative may be given the night before the test. Food is restricted after midnight before the test. Enemas or suppositories are given on the morning of the test to clean the bowel. The barium enema creates a feeling of fullness, and the client will feel the urge to defecate. Test usually lasts 30–45 minutes. There may be some cramping. Special tubes with balloons are often used to help the client retain the barium. The client is asked to assume various positions (e.g., left lateral, then right lateral) Client will probably pass the barium at the x-ray department. | Provide a rest period afterward; the procedure is fatiguing. Encourage fluids to prevent constipation. Observe stool for passage of barium, and assess regularity of bowel movements. Notify primary care provider if barium does not pass in 2–3 days. An enema may be required if client does not pass all the barium. |

I. STUDIES OF THE GALLBLADDER AND BILE DUCTS

Name	Description	Nursing Intervention	
		Preprocedure	Postprocedure
Cholecystography (oral cholecystography)	X-ray films are taken of the gallbladder after a contrast dye has been given orally.	A fat-free supper is given the evening before. Check for allergy to the contrast dye, which contains iodine. A laxative may be given the evening before, or an enema the morning of the test. Six or more contrast pills (e.g., Telepaque) are given in 5-minute intervals the evening before the test, each with 4–6 ounces of water. The client fasts from midnight the evening before but may drink water.	Provide a rest period. Have client resume a regular diet. Provide a snack if the client is hungry. Assess allergy to the contrast dye.

		Explain that (a) a fatty drink may be given during the test, (b) no discomfort is usually felt, and (c) the procedure lasts about 30–45 minutes.	Assess for allergy to the dye.
Intravenous cholangiography	X-ray films are taken of the bile ducts after dye has been administered intravenously.	The client fasts from midnight the evening before the test but may drink water. The bowel is cleaned with a laxative the evening before or with an enema the morning of the test. Check for allergy to iodine contained in the dye. Explain that iodine dye is given intravenously in the x-ray department. A test for allergy is given in the arm before the test.	Observe intravenous site for bleeding, tenderness.

(continued)

I. Studies of the Gallbladder and Bile Ducts 193

I. Studies of the Gallbladder and Bile Ducts (*continued*)

Name	Description	Nursing Intervention	
		Preprocedure	Postprocedure
Percutaneous transhepatic cholangiography	A needle is inserted through the abdominal wall into the biliary radicle, and a contrast agent is injected. Test distinguishes obstructive from nonobstructive jaundice.	Complete study lasts 3–4 hours. See preparation for intravenous cholangiography. Explain that procedure lasts approximately 30 minutes.	Monitor vital signs q15min for 1 hour, q30min for 4 hours, and then q4h until client is stable. Encourage bed rest. Position client on right side to place pressure on the puncture site to prevent bleeding.
Postoperative cholangiography	Dye is injected through the T-tube; x-ray films are taken and fluoroscopy is done to determine whether the common bile duct is unobstructed.	See preparation for intravenous cholangiography.	Monitor puncture site for bleeding. If T-tube is in place, clamp or attach to drainage as ordered. If T-tube is removed, apply sterile dressing.

J. RADIOGRAPHIC STUDIES: INTRAVENOUS PYELOGRAPHY, ANGIOGRAPHY, MYELOGRAPHY

Name	Description	Nursing Intervention	
		Preprocedure	Postprocedure
Intravenous pyelography or urography (IVP, IVU)	An intravenous injection of radiopaque material is given to examine the kidneys and ureters.	A strong laxative (e.g., castor oil) is given the afternoon before the test to clear the bowel of fecal material, which can obstruct the view of the urinary structures. The client fasts from midnight prior to the test. Check for allergy to iodine. Explain that (a) an intravenous injection will be administered in the x-ray department and (b) the procedure lasts about 1 hour.	Encourage fluid intake. The client resumes a regular diet. Provide for rest; the laxative and fasting can cause weakness. Observe for reactions to the radiopaque dye.

(continued)

J. Radiographic Studies: Intravenous Pyelography, Angiography, Myelography (*continued*)

Name	Description	Nursing Intervention	
		Preprocedure	Postprocedure
Angiography, for example, cerebral angiography (vascular system of the brain), coronary arteriography (coronary arteries), renal angiography (vascular system of the kidneys), pulmonary angiography (vascular system of the lungs)	A radiopaque material is injected into an artery or vein to examine portions of the vascular system.	For some of these procedures, a catheter may be inserted into an artery or vein prior to the injection of radiopaque material. Before some procedures, the client is given a sedative. The client fasts from midnight prior to the test. A strong laxative may be given the evening before certain tests (e.g., renal arteriography). Client is tested for allergy to iodine. The time needed for these procedures varies. Some may take up to 3 hours.	Bed rest is generally maintained for up to 12 hours. Monitor the client's radial pulse, respirations, and blood pressure q15–30min until they stabilize. Monitor peripheral pulses distal to the injection site. Observe the injection site for bleeding and swelling. Apply cold pack to prevent swelling. Determine any discomfort experienced by the client.

| Myelography | A contrast material is injected into the subarachnoid space, and x-ray films are taken of the spinal cord, nerve roots, and vertebrae. | Fasting may be required from midnight prior to the test. The client may be given a sedative before the procedure. Explain that (a) a radiopaque oil dye is injected via a lumbar puncture in the x-ray department; (b) the client will assume various positions (e.g., lateral for a lumbar puncture, then prone, and then tilted on x-ray table equipped with shoulder and foot supports); and (c) client may feel some pain when the oil is removed. The pain is due to irritation of the nerve roots. The procedure may last approximately 2 hours. | The client is generally positioned flat in bed for 24 hours to minimize headache and/or nausea; however, client may be positioned with the head elevated above the level of the spine if the dye has not been completely removed. This prevents the dye from moving to the head and causing an inflammation of the meninges (meningitis). Monitor vital signs and neurologic status (e.g., complaints of numbness, pain, or tingling in the extremities; muscle weakness). Monitor urinary output. |

K. KEY INFORMATION ABOUT VITAMINS

	RDA for Healthy Adults Ages 19–50	Major Dietary Sources	Major Functions	Signs of Severe, Prolonged Deficiency	Signs of Extreme Excess
Fat-Soluble Vitamins					
A (retinol)	Females: 800 RE; if lactating, 1200 RE Males: 1000 RE	Fat-containing and fortified dairy products; liver; provitamin carotene in orange and deep green fruits and vegetables	Vision growth; bone development; epithelial tissue formation; cellular differentiation	Night blindness; keratinization of epithelial tissues, including the cornea of the eye (xerophthalmia), causing permanent blindness; dry, scaling skin; increased susceptibility to infection	Preformed vitamin A: damage to liver and bone; dry skin; headache; irritability; vomiting; hair loss; blurred vision Carotenoids: yellowed skin

Vitamin	Recommended amount	Sources	Functions	Deficiency	Toxicity
D (calciferol)	<25 years: 10 µg >25 years: 5 µg	Fortified and full-fat dairy products, fish liver oils, egg yolk (diet often not as important as sunlight exposure)	Promotes absorption and use of calcium and phosphorus	Rickets (bone deformities) in children; osteomalacia (bone softening) in adults	Calcium deposition in tissues leading to cerebral, cardiovascular, and kidney damage
E (tocopherol)	Females: 8 α-tocopherol equivalents Males: 10 α-tocopherol equivalents	Vegetable oils and their products; nuts, seeds	Antioxidant to prevent cell membrane damage	Possible anemia and neurologic effects	Generally nontoxic; may worsen clotting defect in vitamin K deficiency
K	Females: <25:60 µg; >25:65 µg Males: <25:70 µg; >25:80 µg	Green vegetables; green tea	Aids in formation of certain proteins, especially those for blood clotting	Defective blood coagulation causing severe bleeding on injury	Liver damage and anemia from high doses of the synthetic form (menadione)

(continued)

K. Key Information about Vitamins *(continued)*

	RDA for Healthy Adults Ages 19–50	Major Dietary Sources	Major Functions	Signs of Severe, Prolonged Deficiency	Signs of Extreme Excess
Water-Soluble Vitamins					
Thiamin (B₁)	Females: 1.1 mg Males: 1.5 mg	Brewer's yeast, pork, legumes, peanuts, enriched or whole-grain products	Coenzyme used in energy metabolism	Dementia; paralysis; neuropathy; edema; beriberi	Generally nontoxic
Riboflavin (B₂)	Females: 1.3 mg Males: 1.7 mg	Beef liver, dairy products, meats, eggs, enriched grain products	Coenzyme used in energy metabolism	Skin lesions	Generally nontoxic
Niacin	Females: 15 niacin equivalents Males: 19 niacin equivalents	Nuts, meats; provitamin tryptophan in most proteins	Coenzyme used in energy metabolism	Pellagra (multiple vitamin deficiencies, including niacin)	Flushing of face, neck, hands; potential liver damage

B₆ (pyridox-ine)	Females: 1.6 mg Males: 2.0 mg	Coenzyme used in amino acid metabo-lism	Nervous, skin, and muscular disorders; anemia	Ataxia, neuropathy
Folic acid (folate)	Females: 180 μg Males: 200 μg	Coenzyme used in DNA and RNA metabolism; single carbon utilization	Megaloblastic anemia (large, immature red blood cells); gas-trointestinal distur-bances	Generally nontoxic
B₁₂ (cobal-amin)	2 μg	Coenzyme used in DNA and RNA metabolism; single carbon utilization	Megaloblastic anemia; pernicious anemia when due to inade-quate intrinsic factor; nervous system dam-age	Thought to be nontoxic
Pantothenic acid	4–7 mg	Coenzyme used in energy metabolism	None	Generally nontoxic; occa-sionally causes diarrhea
Biotin	30–100 μg	Coenzyme used in energy metabolism	Scaly dermatitis	Thought to be nontoxic

(continued)

K. Key Information about Vitamins (*continued*)

	RDA for Healthy Adults Ages 19–50	Major Dietary Sources	Major Functions	Signs of Severe, Prolonged Deficiency	Signs of Extreme Excess
C (ascorbic acid)	60 mg	Fruits and vegetables, especially broccoli, cabbage, cantaloupe, cauliflower, citrus fruits, green pepper, kiwi fruit, strawberries	Functions in synthesis of collagen; is an antioxidant; aids in detoxification; improves iron absorption; still under intense study	Scurvy; petechiae (minute hemorrhages around hair follicles); weakness; delayed wound healing; impaired immune response	Gastrointestinal upset; interferes with certain lab tests

L. KEY INFORMATION ABOUT MINERALS

Major Mineral	RDA for Healthy Adults Ages 19–50	Major Dietary Sources	Major Functions	Signs of Severe, Prolonged Deficiency	Signs of Extreme Excess
Calcium	1200 mg for ages 19–24; 800 mg for males 25 and older; 1000–1500 mg for females 25 and older	Milk, cheese, dark green vegetables, legumes	Bone and tooth formation; blood clotting; nerve transmission	Stunted growth; perhaps less bone mass; perhaps hypertension	Depressed absorption of some other minerals; perhaps kidney damage
Chloride	*	Same as for sodium	Plays a role in acid–base balance; formation of gastric juice	Muscle cramps; reduced appetite; poor growth	High blood pressure in genetically predisposed individuals
Magnesium	Females: 280 mg Males: 350 mg	Whole grains, green leafy vegetables	Component of enzymes	Neurologic disturbances	Neurologic disturbances
Phosphorus	1200 mg for ages 19–24; 800 mg for 25 and older	Milk, cheese, meat, poultry, whole grains	Bone and tooth formation; acid–base balance; component of coenzymes	Weakness; demineralization of bone	Depressed absorption of some minerals

(continued)

L. Key Information about Minerals (*continued*)

Major Mineral	RDA for Healthy Adults Ages 19–50	Major Dietary Sources	Major Functions	Signs of Severe, Prolonged Deficiency	Signs of Extreme Excess
Potassium	*	Meats, milk, many fruits and vegetables, whole grains	Body water balance; nerve function	Muscular weakness; paralysis	Muscular weakness; cardiac arrest
Sodium	*	Salt, soy sauce, cured meats, pickles, canned soups, processed cheese	Body water balance; nerve function	Muscle cramps; reduced appetite	High blood pressure in genetically predisposed individuals
Sulfur	(Provided by sulfur amino acids)	Sulfur amino acids in dietary proteins	Component of cartilage, tendons, and proteins	Related to protein deficiency	Excess sulfur-containing amino acid intake leads to poor growth; liver damage

*No formal recommendation.

M. KEY INFORMATION ABOUT TRACE MINERALS

Trace Mineral	RDA for Healthy Adults Ages 19–50	Major Dietary Sources	Major Functions	Signs of Severe, Prolonged Deficiency	Signs of Extreme Excess
Chromium	50–200 µg[†]	Brewer's yeast, liver, seafood, meat, potatoes	Involved in glucose and energy metabolism	Impaired glucose metabolism	Lung and kidney damage (occupational exposures only)
Cobalt	(Required as vitamin B₁₂)*	Animal products	Component of vitamin B₁₂	Not reported except as vitamin B₁₂ deficiency	Polycythemia
Copper	1.5–3 mg[†]	Seafood, nuts, legumes, organ meats	Component of enzymes	Anemia; bone and cardiovascular changes	Nausea; liver damage
Fluoride	1.5–4 mg[†]	Drinking water, tea, seafood	Maintenance of tooth (and maybe bone) structure	Higher frequency of tooth decay	Acute: gastrointestinal distress Chronic: mottling of teeth; skeletal deformation

(continued)

M. Key Information about Trace Minerals *(continued)*

Major Mineral	RDA for Healthy Adults Ages 19–50	Major Dietary Sources	Major Functions	Signs of Severe, Prolonged Deficiency	Signs of Extreme Excess
Iodine	150 μg	Fish and shellfish, dairy products, iodized salt, some breads	Component of thyroid hormones	Goiter (enlarged thyroid); mental retardation	Goiter
Iron	Females: 15 mg Males: 10 mg	Meats, eggs, beans, whole grains, green leafy vegetables	Components of hemoglobin, myoglobin, and enzymes	Iron-deficiency anemia; weakness; impaired immune function	Acute: shock; death Chronic: liver damage; cardiac failure
Manganese	2–5 mg†	Nuts, whole grains, vegetables and fruits, tea	Component of enzymes	Abnormal bone and cartilage; sterility	Central nervous system damage (occupational exposures)
Molybdenum	75–250 μg†	Beans, cereals, dark green, leafy vegetables	Component of enzymes	Disorder in nitrogen excretion; mental changes	Inhibition of enzymes; gout-like syndrome

Selenium	Females: 55 µg Males: 70 µg	Seafood, meats, whole grains, Brazil nuts	Component of enzymes; functions in close association with vitamin E	Muscle pain; maybe heart muscle deterioration	Unknown
Zinc	Females: 12 mg Males: 15 mg	Meats, seafood, whole grains	Component of enzymes	Growth failure; scaly dermatitis; reproductive failure; impaired immune function	Acute: nausea; vomiting; diarrhea Chronic: adversely affects copper metabolism and immune function; anemia

*No formal recommendation.
†Estimated safe and adequate daily dietary intake.

Vaccine ▼ / Age ▶	Birth	1 month	2 months	4 months	6 months	12 months	15 months	18 months	24 months	4–6 years	11–12 years	13–14 years	15 years	16–18 years
Hepatitis B[1]	HepB	HepB		HepB[1]		HepB					HepB Series			
Diphtheria, Tetanus, Pertussis[2]			DTaP	DTaP	DTaP		DTaP			DTaP	Tdap		Tdap	
Haemophilus influenzae type b[3]			Hib	Hib	Hib[3]	Hib								
Inactivated Poliovirus			IPV	IPV		IPV				IPV				
Measles, Mumps, Rubella[4]						MMR				MMR	MMR			
Varicella[5]							Varicella				Varicella			
Meningococcal[6]								Vaccines within broken line are for selected populations	MPSV4		MCV4		MCV4	MCV4
Pneumococcal[7]			PCV	PCV	PCV	PCV	PCV		PCV		PPV			
Influenza[8]					Influenza (Yearly)					Influenza (Yearly)				
Hepatitis A[9]									HepA Series					

This schedule indicates the recommended ages for routine administration of currently licensed childhood vaccines, as of December 1, 2005, for children through age 18 years. Any dose not administered at the recommended age should be administered at any subsequent visit when indicated and feasible. ▮ Indicates age groups that warrant special effort to administer those vaccines not previously administered. Additional vaccines may be licensed and recommended during the year. Licensed combination vaccines may be used whenever

any components of the combination are indicated and other components of the vaccine are not contraindicated and if approved by the Food and Drug Administration for that dose of the series. Providers should consult the respective ACIP statement for detailed recommendations. Clinically significant adverse events that follow immunization should be reported to the Vaccine Adverse Event Reporting System (VAERS). Guidance about how to obtain and complete a VAERS form is available at **www.vaers.hhs.gov** or by telephone, **800-822-7967**.

▮ Range of recommended ages   ▮ Catch-up immunization   ▮ 11–12 year old assessment

O. RECOMMENDED ADULT IMMUNIZATION SCHEDULE—UNITED STATES, 2006–2007

Vaccine ▼ / Age group ▶	19–49 years	50–64 years	≥65 years
Tetanus, diphtheria, pertussis (Td/Tdap)[1],*	1 dose Td booster every 10 yrs		
	Substitute 1 dose of Tdap for Td		
Human papillomavirus (HPV)[2]	3 doses (females)		
Measles, mumps, rubella (MMR)[3],*	1 or 2 doses	1 dose	
Varicella[4],*	2 doses (0, 4–8 wks)	2 doses (0, 4–8 wks)	
Influenza[5],*	1 dose annually	1 dose annually	
Pneumococcal (polysaccharide)[6,7]	1–2 doses		1 dose
Hepatitis A[8],*	2 doses (0, 6–12 mos, or 0, 6–18 mos)		
Hepatitis B[9],*	3 doses (0, 1–2, 4–6 mos)		
Meningococcal[10]	1 or more doses		

*Covered by the Vaccine Injury Compensation Program. NOTE: These recommendations must be read with the footnotes (see reverse).

☐ For all persons in this category who meet the age requirements and who lack evidence of immunity (e.g., lack documentation of vaccination or have no evidence of prior infection)

■ Recommended if some other risk factor is present (e.g., on the basis of medical, occupational, lifestyle, or other indications)

(continued)

O. Adult Immunizations   209

O. Recommended Adult Immunization Schedule–United States, 2006–2007 (continued)

Vaccine ▼ / Indication ▲	Pregnancy	Congenital immunodeficiency, leukemia,[11] lymphoma, generalized malignancy, cerebrospinal fluid leaks, therapy with alkylating agents, antimetabolites, radiation, or high-dose, long-term corticosteroids	Diabetes, heart disease, chronic pulmonary disease, chronic alcoholism	Asplenia[11] (including elective splenectomy and terminal complement component deficiencies)	Chronic liver disease, recipients of clotting factor concentrates	Kidney failure, end-stage renal disease, recipients of hemodialysis	Human immunodeficiency virus (HIV) infection[11]	Healthcare workers
Tetanus, diphtheria, pertussis (Td/Tdap)[1,*]	1 dose Td booster every 10 yrs ··· Substitute 1 dose of Tdap for Td ···							
Human papillomavirus (HPV)[2]		3 doses for women through age 26 yrs (0, 2, 6 mos)						
Measles, mumps, rubella (MMR)[3,*]			1 or 2 doses					
Varicella[4,*]			2 doses (0, 4–8 wks)					2 doses
Influenza[5,*]	1 dose annually		1 dose annually	1 dose annually		1 dose annually		
Pneumococcal (polysaccharide)[6,7]	1–2 doses	1–2 doses						1–2 doses
Hepatitis A[8,*]	2 doses (0, 6–12 mos, or 0, 6–18 mos)	2 doses (0, 6–12 mos, or 0, 6–18 mos)	2 doses		2 doses (0, 6–12 mos, or 0, 6–18 mos)			
Hepatitis B[9,*]	3 doses (0, 1–2, 4–6 mos)	3 doses (0, 1–2, 4–6 mos)			3 doses (0, 1–2, 4–6 mos)			
Meningococcal[10]	1 dose	1 dose		1 dose		1 dose		

*Covered by the Vaccine Injury Compensation Program. NOTE: These recommendations must be read with the footnotes (see reverse).

☐ For all persons in this category who meet the age requirements and who lack evidence of immunity (e.g., lack documentation of vaccination or have no evidence of prior infection)

☐ Recommended if some other risk factor is present (e.g., on the basis of medical, occupational, lifestyle, or other indications)

▨ Contraindicated

Approved by
the Advisory Committee on Immunization Practices,
the American College of Obstetricians and Gynecologists,
the American Academy of Family Physicians,

DEPARTMENT OF HEALTH AND HUMAN SERVICES
CENTERS FOR DISEASE CONTROL AND PREVENTION

CDC

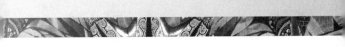

GLOSSARY

abduction movement of a body part away from the midline of the body

abrasion scraping away of the surface of a structure, such as the skin or teeth

abscess a localized collection of pus and disintegrating body cells

absorption (of drug) the process by which a drug passes into the bloodstream

acidosis (acidemia) a condition that occurs with increases in blood carbonic acid or with decreases in blood bicarbonate; arterial blood pH below 7.35

acromion (acromial process) the lateral projection of the scapula extending over the shoulder joint

activities of daily living (ADLs) the tasks of daily life, such as eating, bathing, and dressing

acute sharp or severe; describing a severe condition with a sudden onset and short course (as opposed to chronic)

adduction movement of a body part toward the midline of the body

adipose fat; of a fatty nature

adventitious breath sounds abnormal breath sounds

aldosterone a hormone produced by the adrenal cortex that regulates the level of sodium in the body

alkalosis (alkalemia) a condition that occurs with increases in blood bicarbonate or decreases in blood carbonic acid; arterial blood pH above 7.45

alopecia abnormal loss of hair

ampule a small, sealed glass flask, usually designed to hold a single dose of medication

analgesic a medication used to decrease pain

anaphylaxis (anaphylactic shock, anaphylactic reaction) a severe allergic reaction

anemia a condition in which the blood is deficient in red blood cells or hemoglobin

anesthesia loss of sensation or feeling; induced loss of the sense of pain

aneurysm dilation of the wall of an artery or vein

angiography a diagnostic procedure allowing x-ray visualization of the vascular system after injection of a radiopaque dye

anorexia lack of appetite

anoxia systemic absence or reduction of oxygen in the body tissues below physiologic levels

anterior or at the front of

antibiotic a substance that has the capacity to inhibit the growth of or kill microorganisms

antibody (immunoglobulin) a protective substance produced in the body to counteract antigens

antidiuretic hormone (ADH) a hormone that is stored and released by the posterior pituitary gland and that controls water reabsorption from the kidney tubules; also referred to as *vasopressin*

antigen a substance capable of inducing the formation of antibodies

antipyretic a substance that is effective in reducing fever

antiseptic an agent that inhibits the growth of some microorganisms

anuria the failure of the kidneys to produce urine, resulting in total lack of urination or output of less than 100 mL per day in an adult

aphasia the inability to communicate by speech, signs, or writing, resulting from an injury or disease

apical pulse the central pulse, located at the apex of the heart

apical-radial pulse simultaneous measurement of the apical beat and the radial pulse

apnea cessation of breathing

approximate to bring close together (referring to wound or incision edges)

arrhythmia an irregular cardiac rhythm

arteriosclerosis a condition in which the walls of the arteries become hardened, thickened, and less compliant

ascites the accumulation of fluid in the abdominal cavity

asepsis freedom from infection or infectious material

asphyxia a condition resulting from a lack of oxygen

aspirate to remove gases or fluids from a cavity by using suction

astringent an agent that causes contraction or shrinkage of tissue; usually applied topically

ataxia failure of muscle coordination

atelectasis collapse of lung tissue

atony lack of normal muscle tone

atrophy a wasting away or decrease in size of a cell, tissue, body organ, or muscle

auscultation the practice of examining the body by listening to body sounds

axilla the armpit (plural: axillae)

axillary line an imaginary line extending vertically from the anterior fold of the axilla

bacteriuria bacteria in the urine

barium a metallic element commonly used in solution as a contrast medium for x-ray filming of the gastrointestinal tract

barium enema x-ray filming of the large intestine using a contrast medium; also called a *lower gastrointestinal series*

barium swallow x-ray filming of the esophagus, stomach, and duodenum; also referred to as an *upper gastrointestinal series*

barrel chest a chest shape in which the ratio of the anteroposterior diameter to the lateral diameter is 1 to 1

basal metabolic rate (BMR) the rate of energy utilization in the body required to maintain body functions at rest

bilateral affecting two sides

bilirubin orange or yellow pigment in the bile

binder a type of bandage applied to large body areas, such as the abdomen or chest

biopsy the removal and examination of tissue from the living body

bleb (wheal) a small, smooth, slightly raised area on the skin, usually filled with fluid

brachial pulse a pulse located on the inner side of the biceps muscle just below the axilla; usually palpated medially in the antecubital space

bradycardia an abnormally slow heart rate, below 60 beats per minute in an adult

bronchial sounds normal loud, harsh, hollow blowing sounds heard by auscultation over the trachea and major bronchi

bronchodilator an agent that dilates the bronchi of the lungs

bronchopneumonia an infection that originates in the bronchi and involves patches of lung tissue

bronchoscope a lighted instrument used to visualize the bronchi of the lungs

bronchovesicular sounds combination of bronchial and vesicular sounds heard by auscultation over parts of the chest where a bronchus is near lung tissue

bruxism grinding of the teeth during sleep

buccal pertaining to the cheek

buffer an agent or system that tends to maintain constancy of or that prevents changes in the chemical concentration of a substance

bulimia an uncontrollable compulsion to consume enormous amounts of food and then expel the food by self-induced vomiting or by taking laxatives

calculus a stone composed of minerals that is formed in the body, for example, a renal calculus formed in the kidney

cannula a tube with a lumen (channel), which is inserted into a cavity or duct and is often fitted with a trocar during insertion

canthus the angle formed by the upper and lower eyelids; each eye has an inner and an outer canthus

cardiac arrest the cessation of heart function

cardiac output the amount of blood ejected from the heart per minute by ventricular contraction; it is the stroke volume times the heart rate per minute

cardiopulmonary resuscitation (CPR) artificial stimulation of the heart and lungs; also referred to as *basic life support (BLS)*

caries decay of a tooth or bone

carina the ridge or junction where the main bronchi meet the trachea

carminative an agent that prevents the formation of gas in the colon

carotid arteries major arteries lying on either side of the trachea and larynx

cataract opacity of the lens of the eye or its capsule

cathartic (laxative) a drug that induces evacuation of feces from the large intestine

catheter a tube of plastic, rubber, metal, or other material used to remove or inject fluids into a cavity, such as the bladder

caudal anesthetic an anesthetic injected into the caudal canal, below the spinal cord

cellulitis inflammation of cellular tissue

centigrade (Celsius) a thermometer scale used to measure heat; the freezing point of water is 0°C, and the boiling point is 100°C

central venous pressure (CVP) a measurement of the pressure of the blood, in millimeters of water, within the vena cava or the right atrium of the heart

cephalocaudal proceeding in the direction from head to toe

cerebrospinal fluid fluid contained within the four ventricles of the brain, the subarachnoid space, and the central canal of the spinal cord

cerumen waxlike material found in the external auditory canal

chancre a papular lesion (sore) occurring at the primary site of infection in some diseases; the primary sore of syphilis

Cheyne-Stokes respirations rhythmic waxing and waning of respirations from very deep breathing to very shallow breathing with periods of temporary apnea; often associated with cardiac failure, increased intracranial pressure, or brain damage

chill shivering and shaking of the body with involuntary contractions of the voluntary muscles

cholangiogram an x-ray film of the biliary tract taken after the injection of a dye

cholecystogram an x-ray film of the gallbladder after the ingestion of a contrast dye; also called *oral cholecystography*

cholesterol a lipid that does not contain fatty acid but possesses many of the chemical and physical properties of other lipids

chronic persisting over a long time

chyme semifluid material produced by gastric digestion of food in the stomach; it is found in the small and large intestines

cicatrix scar

cilia hairlike projections from cells, for example, cells of the mucous membrane of the respiratory tract

circulatory overload a state of increased blood volume

circumduction movement of the distal part of a bone in a circle, with the proximal end remaining fixed

clean technique a technique that maintains an area or articles free from infectious agents

closed wound a wound in which there is no break in the skin

clubbing (of nails) an elevation of the proximal aspect of the nail and softening of the nail bed

coagulate to clot

cochlea a tubular structure in the inner ear that contains the organ for hearing

colic paroxysmal intestinal cramplike pain

collagen a protein found in connective tissue; a whitish protein substance that adds tensile strength to a wound

colonoscope a lighted instrument used to visualize the interior of the colon

colostomy an artificial abdominal opening into the colon (large bowel)

comatose a state of unconsciousness in which the person shows no response to maximum painful stimuli, absence of reflexes, and absence of muscle tone in the extremities

commode a portable chairlike structure used as a toilet

communicable disease (infectious disease) a disease that can spread from one person to another

compliance (vascular) distensibility or the ability to contract and expand

congenital existing at, and often before, birth

conjunctiva the delicate membrane that covers the eyeball and lines the eyelids

conjunctivitis inflammation of the conjunctiva

consciousness a person's normal state of awareness of the environment, self, and others

consensual reaction (of the eyes) a reaction in which one pupil constricts quickly in response to a bright light and the other pupil constricts also, but more slowly

constipation passage of small, dry, hard stool or passage of no stool for an abnormally long time

contaminated possessing disease-producing microorganisms

contracture permanent shortening of a muscle and subsequent shortening of tendons and ligaments

contusion a closed wound that occurs as a result of a blow from a blunt instrument; a bruise

core temperature temperature of the deep structures of the body

cornea the transparent covering of the anterior eye that connects with the sclera

costal angle the angle formed between the ribs and the sternum

costal (thoracic) breathing breathing using chiefly the intercostal muscles

costovertebral angle the angle formed by a rib and the spine

counterirritant an agent that produces an irritation with the intent of relieving some other problem

crackles (rales) rattling or bubbling breath sounds generally heard on inspiration

creatinine a nitrogenous waste that is excreted in the urine

Credé's maneuver manual exertion of pressure on the bladder to force urine out

crepitus (crepitation) skeletal: a grating sound caused by bone fragments rubbing together; respiratory: a dry, crackling sound like that of crumpled cellophane, produced by air in the subcutaneous tissue or by air moving through fluid in the alveoli of the lungs

culture in microbiology, the cultivation of microorganisms or cells in a special growth medium

cyanosis bluish discoloration of the skin, nail beds, and mucous membranes, due to reduced oxygen in the blood

cyst an enclosed cavity or sac lined by epithelium and containing liquid or semisolid material

cystitis inflammation of the urinary bladder

cystoscope a lighted instrument used to visualize the interior of the urinary bladder

cystoscopy visual examination of the urinary bladder with a cystoscope

cytology the study of the origin, structure, function, and pathology of cells

debride to remove foreign and dying tissue from a wound so that healthy tissue is exposed

defecation expulsion of feces from the rectum and anus

dehiscence a splitting open or rupture

dehydration insufficient fluid in the body

dementia decline in memory and other cognitive abilities

dependent edema edema that collects in the lower parts of the body, where hydrostatic pressure is greatest

dermatitis inflammation of the skin

dermatologic preparation a medication applied to the skin

dermis (corium) true skin, containing blood vessels, nerves, hair follicles, and glands

detrusor muscle the three layers of smooth muscle that make up the urinary bladder

dextrose a sugar; also called *glucose*

diagnosis a statement or conclusion concerning the nature of some phenomenon

diaphoresis profuse sweating

diaphragmatic (abdominal) breathing breathing that chiefly involves movement of the diaphragm and the abdomen

diarrhea defecation of liquid feces and increased frequency of defecation

diastole the period when the ventricles of the heart are relaxed

diastolic pressure the pressure of the blood against the arterial walls when the ventricles of the heart are at rest

digital performed with the finger

disorientation a state of mental confusion; loss of bearings, time, and place

distal farthest from the point of reference

diuresis see *polyuria*

diuretic an agent that increases the production of urine

dorsal of, toward, or at the back

dorsal flexion movement of the ankle so that the toes point up

dorsalis pedis pulse a pulse located on the instep of the foot

dorsal recumbent position a back-lying position with the head and shoulders slightly elevated

drainage a discharge from a wound or cavity

drug interaction the beneficial or harmful interaction of one drug with another drug

drug tolerance a condition in which successive increases in the dosage of a drug are required to maintain a given therapeutic effect

drug toxicity the quality of a drug that exerts a deleterious effect on an organism or tissue

dullness (in percussion) decreased resonance or percussion sound that occurs over dense tissue or large amounts of fluid

dysmenorrhea painful menstruation

dyspepsia indigestion

dysphagia difficulty or inability to swallow

dysphasia difficulty speaking

dysphoria a feeling of disquiet, restlessness, anxiety, depression

dyspnea difficult and labored breathing in which the client has a persistent unsatisfied need for air

dysrhythmia an irregular cardiac rhythm

dysuria painful or difficult urination

ecchymosis a blotchy area of discoloration of the skin; a bruise

edema excess interstitial fluid

electrocardiogram (ECG, EKG) a graph of the electric activity of the heart

electroencephalogram (EEG) a graph of the electric activity of the brain

electrolyte ionized salts found in cells, tissue fluids, and blood

embolus a blood clot (or a substance, such as air) that has moved from its place of origin and is obstructing the circulation in a blood vessel (plural: emboli)

emollient an agent that soothes and softens skin or mucous membrane; often an oily substance

emphysema a chronic obstructive lung disorder in which the terminal bronchioles become distended and plugged with mucus

emulsion a preparation in which one liquid is distributed throughout another

endogenous developing from within

endoscope a lighted instrument used to visualize the interior of a hollow organ

endothelium the layer of endothelial cells lining the blood vessels, cavities of the heart, and serous cavities

endotracheal tube a tube inserted into the trachea

enema a solution injected into the rectum and the sigmoid colon

enteric referring to the small intestines

enteric coated surrounded with a special coating used for tablets and capsules that prevents release of the drug until it is in the intestines

enteric feeding a feeding administered directly into the small intestine through a tube

enterostomal therapist a person who specializes in ostomy care

enzyme a biologic catalyst that induces chemical reactions

epidemic the occurrence of a disease in many people at the same time or in rapid succession in an area

epidermis the outermost, nonvascular layer of skin

epistaxis nosebleed

eructation ejection of gas from the stomach (belching)

erythema redness that is associated with a variety of rashes

erythrocyte red blood cell

eschar a slough of dried plasma proteins and dead cells; often produced by a burn, corrosive application, or gangrene

esophagoscopy visual examination of the interior of the esophagus with a lighted instrument

etiology cause

eupnea normal respiration that is quiet, rhythmic, and effortless

evisceration removal of or spilling out of the internal organs

exanthema skin rash

excise to cut off or out

excoriation abrasion of the superficial layers of the skin

excretion elimination of waste products from the body

exogenous developing from without

expectorate to cough and spit up mucus or other materials

expiratory reserve volume the maximum amount of air exhaled after a normal exhalation

extension increasing the angle of a joint (between two bones); the act of straightening

external cardiac massage rhythmic massage of the heart muscle over the sternum

extracellular outside the cells

extracellular fluid (ECF) fluid found outside the body cells

extravasation the escape of blood from a vessel into body tissues

exudate material, such as fluid and cells, that has escaped from blood vessels and is deposited in tissues or on tissue surfaces during the inflammatory process

febrile pertaining to a fever; feverish

fecal impaction a mass of hardened feces in the rectum

fecal incontinence inability to control the passage of feces through the anus

feces (stool) body wastes and undigested food eliminated from the rectum

femoral pulse the pulse found in the groin at the midpoint of the inguinal ligament

fever elevated body temperature

fibrillation involuntary contractions of a muscle; cardiac arrhythmia characterized by extremely rapid, irregular, and ineffective contractions of the atria or ventricles

first intention healing primary healing of a wound, which occurs when the tissue surfaces have been approximated

fistula an abnormal communication or passage, usually between two organs or between an organ and the body surface

flaccid weak or lax

flaccid paralysis impaired muscle function with loss of muscle tone

flail chest a condition of the chest wall caused by two or more rib fractures resulting in paradoxical breathing

flatness (in percussion) absence of resonance; extreme dullness

flatulence the presence of excessive amounts of gas in the stomach or intestines

flatus gas or air normally present in the stomach or intestines

flexion decreasing the angle of a joint (between two bones); the act of bending

flowsheet a record used to chart the progress of specific or specialized data, such as vital signs, fluid balance, or routine medications

fluoroscope a device for examining internal structures using roentgen (x-) rays

flushing (of the skin) transient redness of the skin, often of the face and neck; it may be generalized or restricted to a particular area

footdrop plantar flexion of the foot with permanent contracture of the gastrocnemius (calf) muscle and tendon

forceps an instrument with two blades and a handle used to grasp sterile supplies and to compress or grasp tissues

foreskin a covering fold of skin over the glans of the penis; also called the *prepuce*

formulary a collection or list of prescriptions and formulas

Fowler's position a bed-sitting position with the head of the bed raised to 45 degrees

fracture a break in the continuity of bone

fremitus vibration perceptible on palpation

frenulum a fold of mucous membrane that attaches the tongue to the floor of the mouth; a fold on the lower surface of the glans penis that connects it with the prepuce

friction rub see *pleural rub*

gait the way a person walks

gastric pertaining to the stomach

gastrocolic reflex increased peristalsis of the colon after food has entered the stomach

gastroenteritis inflammation of the stomach and the intestines

gastroscopy visual examination of the stomach with a gastroscope

gastrostomy a surgical opening that leads through the abdomen directly into the stomach

gauge (of a needle) the diameter of the shaft of a needle

gavage administration of nourishment to the stomach through a nasogastric or orogastric tube; tube feeding

generic name a drug name not protected by trademark and usually describing the chemical structure of the drug

gingivitis inflammation of the gums

glans penis the cap-shaped, expansive structure at the end of the penis

glaucoma an eye disease characterized by an increase in intraocular pressure that produces changes in the optic disc and the field of vision

glomerular filtrate fluid formed in the nephron of the kidney that is similar to plasma in composition; the precursor of urine

glossitis inflammation of the tongue

glottis the vocal apparatus of the larynx

glucose a monosaccharide occurring in food

glycogen the chief carbohydrate stored in the body, particularly in the liver and muscles

glycosuria the presence of glucose in the urine; glucosuria

gonorrhea a sexually transmitted disease due to Neisseria gonorrhoeae infection

gout a condition characterized by excessive uric acid in the blood

granulation tissue young connective tissue with new capillaries formed in the wound-healing process

half-life (of drug) the time interval required for the body's elimination processes to reduce the concentration of the drug in the body by one half

halitosis bad breath

hallux valgus bunion or lateral deviation of the big toe

Heimlich maneuver subdiaphragmatic abdominal thrusts used to clear an obstructed airway

hemangioma a large, persistent, bright red or dark purple vascular area of the skin

hematemesis the vomiting of blood

hematocrit the percentage of red blood cell mass in proportion to whole blood

hematoma a collection of blood in a tissue, organ, or body space due to a break in the wall of a blood vessel

hematuria the presence of blood in the urine

hemiplegia the loss of movement on one side of the body

hemoglobin the red pigment in red blood cells that carries oxygen

hemoglobinuria the presence of hemoglobin in the urine

hemolysis rupture of red blood cells

hemopneumothorax a collection of blood and air or gas in the pleural cavity

hemoptysis the presence of blood in the sputum

hemorrhage bleeding; the escape of blood from the blood vessels

hemorrhoids distended veins in the anus and rectum

hemothorax a collection of blood in the pleural cavity

heparin a substance that prevents coagulation of blood

heparin lock an indwelling intravenous catheter attached to a sealed injection tip

hernia protrusion of an organ or tissue through an opening in the wall of the cavity that usually contains it

hesitancy (of urination) delay and difficulty initiating voiding

high Fowler's position a bed-sitting position in which the head of the bed is elevated 90 degrees

hirsutism abnormal hairiness, particularly in women

Homans' sign calf pain produced by dorsiflexion of the foot, an early sign of venous thrombosis

homeostasis tendency of the body to maintain a state of balance or equilibrium while continually changing

humidifier a device that adds water vapor to inspired air

hydration the addition of water to a substance or tissue

hydrocephalus a disease process resulting in excessive cerebrospinal fluid within the ventricles of the brain

hydrocortisone an adrenocorticosteroid produced by the adrenal glands or produced synthetically; also called *cortisol*

hyperalgesia extreme sensitivity to pain

hyperalimentation see *total parenteral nutrition*

hypercalcemia excessive calcium in the blood plasma

hypercalciuria excessive calcium in the urine

hypercarbia (hypercapnia) accumulation of carbon dioxide in the blood

hyperemia increased blood flow to an area

hyperextension further extension between two bones or stretching out of a joint

hyperglycemia an increased concentration of glucose in the blood

hyperhidrosis excessive perspiration

hyperkalemia excessive potassium in the blood

hyperlipidemia elevated concentration of lipids in the plasma

hypermagnesemia excessive magnesium in the blood plasma

hypernatremia an elevated level of sodium in the blood plasma

hyperplasia an abnormal increase in the number of normal cells in a tissue or an organ

hyperpnea an increase in the rate of breathing or an increase in depth of respirations

hyperpyrexia an extremely elevated body temperature

hyperreflexia an exaggeration of the reflexes

hyperresonance a sound that is lower-pitched than resonance; booming sound

hypersensitivity an exaggerated response of the body to a foreign substance

hypersomnia excessive sleep

hypertension an abnormally high blood pressure

hyperthermia an abnormally high body temperature, sometimes induced as a therapeutic measure

hypertonicity excessive muscle tone or activity

hypertonic solution a fluid possessing a greater concentration of solutes than plasma

hypertrophy an increase in size of a cell, tissue, or body organ, such as a muscle

hyperventilation an increase in the amount of air entering the lungs, characterized by deep, rapid breaths

hypervolemia an abnormal increase in the body's blood volume; circulatory overload

hypnotic (drug) a drug that induces sleep

hypoalbuminemia reduction in the level of albumin in the blood

hypocalcemia decreased calcium in the blood plasma

hypoglycemia a reduced amount of glucose in the blood

hypokalemia potassium deficit in the blood plasma

hypomagnesemia low magnesium in the blood plasma

hyponatremia an abnormally low amount of sodium in the blood plasma

hypoproteinemia decreased amount of protein in the blood plasma

hypostatic pneumonia an infection of lung tissue resulting from poor circulation or stagnation of secretions

hypotension an abnormally low blood pressure

hypothermia an abnormally low body temperature

hypotonicity decreased muscle tone

hypotonic solution a fluid possessing a lesser concentration of solutes than plasma

hypoventilation a reduction in the amount of air entering the lungs, characterized by shallow respirations

hypovolemia decreased blood volume

hypovolemic shock a state of shock due to a reduction in the volume of circulating blood

hypoxemia low partial pressure of oxygen or low saturation of oxyhemoglobin in the arterial blood

hypoxia oxygen deficiency

iatrogenic caused by the physician or medical therapy

ileal conduit method of diverting urinary flow into a piece of ileum

ileostomy an artificial abdominal opening into the ileum (small bowel)

immobility prescribed or unavoidable restriction of movement in any area of a person's life

immunity a specific resistance of the body to infection; it may be naturally endowed resistance or resistance developed after exposure to a disease agent

immunization the process of becoming immune or rendering someone immune

immunoglobulin a part of the body's plasma proteins; also called *immune bodies* or *antibodies*

impaction a condition of being firmly wedged or lodged; in reference to feces, a collection of hardened puttylike feces in the folds of the rectum

incentive spirometer (sustained maximal inspiration [SMI] device) a device that measures the flow of air through a mouthpiece as the client practices maximal depth of respiration

incision a cut or wound that is intentionally made, for example, during surgery

incompatibility (of drug) undesired chemical or physical reaction between a drug and an infusion solution, between two or more drugs, or between a drug and the container or tubing

incontinence inability to control the elimination of urine (enuresis) or feces (fecal incontinence)

incubation period the time between the entry of microorganisms into the body and the onset of symptoms of the infection

induration hardening

infarct a localized area of necrosis (dead cells) usually caused by obstructed arterial blood flow to the part

infection the disease process produced by microorganisms

infiltration the diffusion or deposition of substances into a tissue

inflammation local and nonspecific defensive tissue response to injury or destruction of cells

infusion the introduction of fluid into a vein or part of the body

inhalation (aerosol) therapy delivery of droplets of medication or moisture suspended in a gas, such as oxygen, by inhalation through the nose or mouth

insomnia inability to initiate or maintain a sufficient quality or quantity of sleep

inspection visual examination to detect features perceptible to the eye

instillation application of a medication into a body cavity or orifice

insulin a hormone secreted by the beta cells of the islands of Langerhans in the pancreas

integument the skin or covering of the body

intercostal between the ribs

intercostal retractions indrawing between the ribs with inspiration

internal rotation a turning toward the midline, such as rotation of the hip joint

interstitial between the cells of the body's tissues

interstitial fluid fluid surrounding the body cells

intestinal distention stretching and inflation of the intestines due to the presence of air or gas

intracellular within a cell or cells

intracellular fluid (cellular fluid, ICF) fluid found within the body cells

intractable pain pain that is resistant to cure or relief

intradermal (intracutaneous) within the skin

intramuscular within or inside muscle tissue

intraoperative period the time during surgery

intrapleural within the pleural cavity

intrathecal within or into the spinal canal

intravascular within a blood vessel

intravenous within a vein

intravenous cholangiogram an x-ray film of the bile ducts after a contrast dye has been administered intravenously

intravenous push (IVP, bolus) direct intravenous administration of a medication

intravenous pyelogram an x-ray film of the kidneys taken after intravenous injection of a radiopaque dye

intravenous pyelography (IVP) x-ray filming of the kidney and ureters after injection of a radiopaque material intravenously; also called *intravenous urography*

intravertebral (intraspinal) within the vertebrae

intubation insertion of a tube

inversion a turning inward

ion an atom with an electric charge

iron-deficiency anemia form of anemia caused by an inadequate supply of iron for synthesis of hemoglobin

irradiation exposure to penetrating rays, such as x-rays, gamma rays, infrared rays, or ultraviolet rays

irrigation (lavage) the washing of a body cavity or a wound

irritant a substance that stimulates unpleasant responses, that is, irritates

ischemia lack of blood supply to a body part

isolation practice that prevents the spread of infection and communicable diseases

isometric having the same measure or length

isotonic having the same tonicity as the body fluids; the term is used to compare solutions of the same strength or concentration

jaundice a yellowish tinge to the skin and mucous membrane caused by excess bilirubin in the blood

jejunum the portion of the small intestine that extends from the duodenum to the ileum

Kardex a portable card index file that organizes data about clients in a concise way and, often, contains nursing care plans

Kegel's exercises exercises for tightening pelvic floor or perineal muscles

ketosis a condition in which excessive ketones are accumulated in the body

Korotkoff's sounds a series of five sounds heard when auscultating blood pressure; these sounds are produced by blood within the artery with each ventricular contraction

kyphosis an exaggerated convexity in the thoracic region of the vertebral column, resulting in a stooped posture

labored breathing difficult or dyspneic breathing

lacerate to tear, rather than cut, a body tissue

lacrimal sac the opening connecting the tear ducts in the inner canthus of the eye to the nasolacrimal duct, which empties into the nasal cavity

lacrimation the secretion and discharge of tears

laryngeal stridor a harsh, crowing sound heard during expiration when a laryngeal obstruction is present

laryngoscopy visual examination of the larynx with a laryngoscope

laryngospasm spasmodic closure of the larynx

lateral to the side, away from the midline

lateral position a side-lying position

lavage an irrigation or washing of a body organ, such as the stomach

laxative a medication that stimulates bowel activity

lentigo senilis clusters of melanocytes that appear as brown "age" spots

lesion the traumatic or pathologic interruption of a tissue or the loss of function of a body part

lethargy drowsiness; a state in which a person sleeps much of the time when the person is not stimulated

leukocyte a white blood cell

leukocytosis an increase in the number of white blood cells

Levin tube a single-lumen nasogastric tube

ligament a broad, fibrous band that holds two or more bones together

liniment a topical liquid applied to the skin frequently to stimulate circulation or to relieve pain

lithotomy position a back-lying position in which the feet are supported in stirrups

lobar pneumonia an infectious disease of one or more lobes of the lung

lobe a well-defined portion of an organ, for example, of the lung or brain

lordosis an exaggerated concavity in the lumbar region of the vertebral column

lumbar puncture (LP, spinal tap) the insertion of a needle into the subarachnoid space at the lumbar region

lumen a channel within a tube, such as the channel of an artery in which blood flows

lung compliance expansibility of the lung

lung recoil the tendency of lungs to collapse away from the chest wall

lymphatic referring to lymph or lymph vessels

maceration the wasting away or softening of a solid as if by the action of soaking

malaise a general feeling of being unwell or indisposed

malignancy abnormal tissue with a tendency to grow and invade other tissues

malleolus a rounded prominence on the distal end of the tibia or fibula

malnutrition a disorder of nutrition; insufficient nourishment of the body cells

mammography x-ray study of breast tissues

mastectomy surgical removal of the breast

masticate to chew

meatus an opening, passage, or channel

medial toward the middle or midline

medical asepsis practices that limit the number, growth, and spread of microorganisms; clean technique

melanin the dark pigment of the skin

meniscus the crescent-shaped structure of the surface of a column of liquid; the crescent-shaped cartilage in the knee joint

metabolism the sum of all the physical and chemical processes by which living substance is formed and maintained and by which energy is made available for use by the organism

metacarpal referring to the part of the hand between the wrist and fingers

micturate (urinate, void) to pass urine from the body

midclavicular line an imaginary line that runs inferiorly and vertically from the center of the clavicle

midsternal line an imaginary line that runs vertically through the middle of the sternum

miosis constriction of the pupil

MMR combined measles, mumps, and rubella vaccine

mons pubis a pillow of adipose tissue situated over the symphysis pubis and covered by coarse hair; also called the *mons veneris*

Montgomery straps tie tapes used to hold dressings in place

morbidity incidence of disease

mucolytic destroying or dissolving mucus

mucous membrane epithelial tissue that lines passages and cavities communicating with the air

mucus a viscous fluid secreted by the mucous membranes

murmur (cardiac) abnormal sounds heard on auscultation of the heart resulting from turbulent blood flow during systole and diastole

mydriatic a medication that dilates the pupils

myelogram an x-ray film of the spinal cord, nerve roots, and vertebrae after injection of a contrast media into the subarachnoid space

myocardial infarction cardiac tissue necrosis resulting from obstruction of the blood flow to the heart

myocardium the heart muscle; the middle layer of the heart tissue

narcotic antagonist a drug that prevents or reverses the action of a narcotic

nasogastric tube a plastic or rubber tube inserted through the nose into the stomach

nasopharynx the upper part of the pharynx adjoining the nasal passage

nausea the urge to vomit

nebulizer an atomizer or sprayer

necrosis death of cells or tissue in contact with living cells

negative nitrogen balance a nitrogen output that exceeds nitrogen intake (related to protein balance)

neoplasm any growth that is new and abnormal

nephritis inflammation of a kidney

nephron the functional unit of the kidney

nephrosis a disease of the kidney in which there is degeneration of kidney function without inflammation; also called *nephrotic syndrome*

nerve block chemical interruption of a nerve pathway effected by injecting a local anesthetic

neurologic pertaining to the nervous system

nocturia (nycturia) increased frequency of urination at night

nocturnal enuresis involuntary urination at night

nonproductive cough a dry, harsh cough without secretions

normal saline an isotonic concentration of salt (NaCl) solution

nosocomial referring to or originating in a hospital or similar institution, as in a nosocomial infection

obesity weight that is 20% greater than the ideal for height and frame

objective data client information that can be determined by observation or measurement by laboratory studies or other means and that can be tested against an accepted standard

obturator anything that obstructs or closes an opening; the obturator of a tracheostomy set fits inside and closes off the end of the outer tube

ointment a semisolid preparation applied externally to the body

olfactory referring to the sense of smell

oliguria production of abnormally small amounts of urine by the kidneys

operative (intraoperative) period the time during surgery

ophthalmoscope an instrument used to examine the interior of the eye

opportunistic pathogen microorganism that causes disease only in a susceptible person

orientation awareness of time, place, and person

orifice an external opening of a body cavity; for example, the anus is the orifice of the large intestine

oropharynx the part of the pharynx that lies between the upper aspect of the epiglottis and the soft palate

orthopnea the ability to breathe only in the upright position, that is, sitting or standing

orthostatic hypotension decrease in blood pressure that occurs on assuming a sitting or standing position

osteoarthritis noninflammatory degenerative joint disease

osteoporosis decrease in bone density; demineralization of bone

ostomy a suffix denoting the formation of an opening or outlet

otoscope an instrument used to inspect the eardrum and external ear canal

outward rotation a turning away from the midline

overweight weight that is 10% greater than the ideal for height and frame

packing filling an open wound or cavity with a material such as gauze

PaCO$_2$ partial pressure of carbon dioxide (arterial blood)

palate the roof of the mouth

palliative affording relief without curing

pallor absence of normal skin color; a whitish-grayish tinge

palpation the act of feeling with the hands, usually the fingers

pandemic an epidemic disease that is widespread

PaO$_2$ partial pressure of oxygen (arterial blood)

papule a small, superficial, round elevation of the skin

paracentesis the insertion of a needle into a cavity (usually the abdominal cavity) to remove fluid

paradoxical breathing the ballooning out of the chest wall during expiration and depression or sucking inward of the chest wall during inspiration

paralysis the impairment or loss of motor function of a body part

paraplegia paralysis of the lower part of the body (including the legs) affecting both motor function and sensation

parasites plants or animals that live on or within another living organism

parenchyma the functional or essential elements of an organ

parenteral accomplished by a needle; occurring outside the alimentary tract; injected into the body through some route other than the alimentary canal, for example, intravenously

paresis partial or incomplete paralysis

paresthesia an abnormal sensation of numbness, burning, or prickling

paronychia inflammation of the tissue surrounding the nail

parotitis (parotiditis) inflammation of the parotid salivary gland

passive exercise exercise during which the muscles do not contract and the nurse, therapist, or client supplies the energy to move the client's body part

paste a semisolid dermatologic preparation that is applied externally

patent open, unobstructed, not closed

pathogen a microorganism capable of producing disease

PCO_2 partial pressure of carbon dioxide

peak plasma level (of drug) the concentration of a drug in the blood plasma that occurs when the elimination rate equals the rate of absorption

pediculosis infestation with lice

penetrating wound a wound created by an instrument that penetrated the skin or mucous membranes deeply into the tissues

Penrose drain a flexible rubber drain

percussion an assessment method in which the body surface is tapped or struck to elicit sound or vibrations from the body structures below the struck area

percutaneous electric stimulation stimulation of major peripheral nerves by electricity applied to the skin surface

perfusion passage of fluid through the vessels of an organ or tissue

perineum the area between the anus and the genitals

perioperative period the time before, during, and after an operation

periorbital around the eye socket

peripheral at the edge or outward boundary

peripheral pulse a pulse located in the periphery of the body

peristalsis wavelike movements produced by circular and longitudinal muscle fibers of the intestinal walls; it propels the intestinal contents onward

peristomal referring to the skin area that surrounds a stoma

peritoneal cavity the area between the layers of peritoneum in the abdomen; a potential space

peritoneum the membrane lining the abdominal walls

peritonitis inflammation of the peritoneum

perspiration the fluid secreted by the sweat glands for excreting waste products and cooling the body

petechiae pinpoint blood vessels visible on the skin

pH a measure of the relative alkalinity or acidity of a solution; a measure of the concentration of hydrogen ions

phalanx any bone of the fingers or toes (plural: phalanges)

phantom pain pain that remains after the perceived location has been removed, such as pain perceived in a foot after the leg has been amputated

phlebitis inflammation of a vein

phlebotomy opening a vein to remove blood

photosensitive sensitive to light

pitch the quality of sound based on the number of vibrations per second or the frequency of vibrations

pitting edema edema in which firm finger pressure on the skin produces an indentation (pit) that remains for several seconds

plantar flexion movement of the ankle so that the toes point downward

plasma the fluid portion of the blood in which the blood cells are suspended

pleural rub (friction rub) a coarse, leathery, or grating sound produced by the rubbing together of the pleura

pneumonia inflammation of the lung tissue

pneumothorax accumulation of air or gas in the pleural cavity

PO$_2$ partial pressure of oxygen (venous blood)

polydipsia excessive thirst

polyneuritis inflammation of many nerves

polyuria (diuresis) the production of abnormally large amounts of urine by the kidneys

popliteal referring to the posterior aspect of the knee

port an opening or entrance

posterior toward, or at the back of

postoperative (postsurgical) period the time following surgery

postural drainage drainage of secretions from various lung segments by the use of specific positions and gravity

precordium the area of the chest over the heart or lower thorax

preoperative period the time before an operation

prepuce see *foreskin*

primary intention healing wound healing that involves minimal or no tissue loss and in which there is minimal granulation tissue and scarring; also referred to as *primary union* or *first intention healing*

proctoscopy visualization of the interior of the rectum with a proctoscope

prodromal period the time from the onset of nonspecific symptoms to the appearance of specific symptoms

prognosis the medical opinion about the outcome of a disease

pronation turning the palm downward; moving the bones of the forearm so that the palm of the hand turns from anterior to posterior in the anatomic position

prone (prone position) lying on the abdomen with the face turned to one side

prophylaxis preventive treatment; prevention of disease

prostatectomy the removal of the prostate gland

prosthesis an artificial part, such as a glass eye, an artificial leg, or dentures

proteinuria the presence of protein in the urine

protocol written plan specifying the procedures to be followed in a particular situation

proximal closest to the point of attachment

pruritus intense itching

ptosis an eyelid that lies at or below the pupil margin; drooping

pulmonary embolus a blood clot that has moved to the lungs

pulse the wave of blood within an artery that is created by contraction of the left ventricle of the heart

pulse deficit a difference between the apical and the radial pulses

pulse pressure the difference between the systolic and the diastolic pressures

pulse rate the number of pulse beats per minute

pulse rhythm the pattern of pulse beats and of intervals between beats

pulse volume the force of the blood with each beat produced by contraction of the left ventricle; pulse strength

puncture (stab) wound a wound made by a sharp instrument penetrating the skin and underlying tissues

purulent containing pus

pus a thick liquid associated with inflammation and composed of cells, liquid, microorganisms, and tissue debris

pustule a small elevation of the skin or mucous membrane, or a clogged pore or follicle containing pus

putrid rotten

pyelogram an x-ray film of the kidney and ureter, showing the pelvis of the kidney

pyrexia elevated body temperature; fever

pyuria the presence of pus in the urine

quality (of sound) subjective description of a sound (e.g., whistling, gurgling, or snapping)

radial pulse the pulse point located where the radial artery passes over the radius of the arm

radiating pain pain perceived at the source and in surrounding or nearby structures

rales see *crackles*

range of motion (ROM) the degree of movement possible for each joint

rebound phenomenon (thermal) the time when the maximum therapeutic effect of a hot or cold application is achieved and the opposite effect begins

reconstitution the technique of adding a solvent to a powdered drug to prepare it for injection

referred pain pain perceived to be in one area but whose source is in another area

reflex an involuntary activity in response to a stimulus

reflux backward flow

regeneration the replacement of destroyed tissue cells by cells that are identical or similar in structure and function

regurgitation the spitting up or backward flow of undigested food

rehabilitation the restoration of a person who is ill or injured to the highest possible functional capacity

renal relating to the kidney

renal dialysis a process in which blood flows from an artery through an artificial membrane that removes impurities; the blood then returns to the client through a vein

renal pelvis the funnel-shaped upper end of each ureter

residual urine the amount of urine remaining in the bladder after a person voids

residual volume (air) the amount of air remaining in the lungs after a person exhales both tidal and expiratory reserve volumes

resonance a low-pitched, hollow sound produced over normal lung tissue when the chest is percussed

respiration the act of breathing; transport of oxygen from the atmosphere to the body cells and transport of carbon dioxide from the cells to the atmosphere

respiratory acidosis (hypercapnia) a state of excess carbon dioxide in the body

respiratory arrest the sudden cessation of breathing

resuscitate to restore life; to revive

retching the involuntary attempt to vomit without producing vomitus

retention (urinary) the accumulation of urine in the bladder and the inability of the bladder to empty itself

retrograde pyelogram an x-ray film taken after a contrast medium is injected through ureteral catheters into the kidneys

retroperitoneal behind the peritoneum

reverse isolation (barrier technique) measures used to prevent certain clients, such as those with severe burns, from coming in contact with microorganisms

reverse Trendelenburg's position a position with the head of the bed raised and the foot lowered, while the bed foundation remains even

Rh factor antigens present on the surface of some people's erythrocytes; persons who possess this factor are referred to as Rh positive, whereas those who do not are referred to as Rh negative

rhinitis inflammation of the mucous membrane of the nose

rhonchi coarse, dry, wheezy, or whistling sounds, more audible during exhalation as the air moves through tenacious mucus or a constricted bronchus

roentgenogram a film produced by photography with x-rays

rotation turning a bone around its central axis either toward the midline of the body (internal rotation) or away from the midline of the body (external rotation)

Salem sump tube a double-lumen nasogastric tube

sanguineous bloody

sanguineous exudate an exudate containing large amounts of red blood cells

saphenous vein either of two superficial veins of the legs; the greater one extends from the foot to the inguinal region, whereas the lesser one extends from the foot up the back of the leg to the knee joint

scar (cicatrix) tissue dense fibrous tissue derived from granulation tissue

sclerosis a process of hardening that occurs from inflammation and disease of the interstitial substance; the term is used to describe hardening of nervous tissues and arterioles

scoliosis a lateral curvature of a part of the vertebral column

sebaceous gland a gland of the dermis that secretes sebum

seborrheic dermatitis a chronic disease of the skin, characterized by scaling and crusted patches on various body areas, such as the scalp

secondary intention healing wound healing that involves the formation of extensive granulation tissue and in which the repair time is lengthy and scarring is extensive

secretion the product of a gland; for example, saliva is the secretion of the salivary glands

sedative an agent that tends to calm or tranquilize

semi-Fowler's position a bed-sitting position in which the head of the bed is elevated at least 30 degrees, with or without knee flexion; also referred to as low-Fowler's position

sensitivity quick response, often referring to the response of microorganisms to an antibiotic

septic referring to a disease process produced by microorganisms or to their poisonous products in the blood

serosanguineous composed of serum and blood

serous exudate a watery exudate composed mainly of serum

serum (blood) blood plasma from which the fibrinogen has been separated during clotting

shock acute circulatory failure

Sickle cell scythe shaped erythrocytes; common to Mediterranean and African populations

side effect an unintended action or complication of a drug

sigmoidoscopy examination of the interior of the sigmoid colon with a sigmoidoscope

sitz bath (hip bath) bath used to soak a client's pelvic or perineal area

sleep apnea periodic cessation of breathing during sleep

smear material spread across a glass slide in preparation for microscopic study

spasm involuntary contraction of a muscle or muscle group

specific gravity the weight or degree of concentration of a substance compared with the weight of an equal amount of another substance used as a standard; for example, water used as a standard has a specific gravity of 1, whereas urine in comparison has a specific gravity of 1.010 to 1.025

speculum a funnel-shaped instrument used to widen and examine canals of the body, such as the vagina or nasal canal

sphincter a ringlike muscle that opens or closes a natural orifice (e.g., the urethra) when it relaxes or contracts

sphygmomanometer an instrument used to measure the pressure of the blood in the arteries

spirometry the measurement of pulmonary volumes and capacities using a spirometer

splint a rigid bar or appliance used to stabilize a body part

sprain injury of the ligaments and associated structure of a joint by wrenching or twisting; associated structures include tendons, muscles, nerves, and blood vessels

sputum the mucous secretion from the lungs, bronchi, and trachea that is expectorated through the mouth

stasis stagnation or stoppage of flow of body fluids, such as intestinal fluids, urine, or blood

stenosis constriction or narrowing of a body canal, vessel, or opening

sterile free from microorganisms, including spores

sterile technique see *surgical asepsis*

sterilization a process that destroys all microorganisms, including spores; causing inability to reproduce

stertor snoring or sonorous respiration, usually due to a partial obstruction of the upper airway

stethoscope an instrument used to listen to various sounds inside the body, such as the heartbeat

stoma an artificial opening; it may be permanent or temporary

stool (feces) waste products excreted from the large intestine

stopcock a valve that controls the flow of fluid or air through a tube

strain (of a muscle) overexertion or overstretching of a muscle or part of a muscle

stridor a shrill, harsh, crowing sound made on inhalation; due to constriction of the upper airway or laryngeal obstruction

stroke volume the amount of blood ejected from the heart with each ventricular contraction

stupor a condition of partial or nearly complete unconsciousness; stuporous clients are never fully awakened even when painfully stimulated

stylet a metal or plastic probe inserted into a needle or cannula to render it stiff and to prevent occlusion of the lumen by particles of tissue

subcostal below the ribs

subcutaneous (hypodermic) beneath the layers of the skin

subjective data client information that only the client can give, such as thoughts or feelings

sublingual under the tongue

suborbital beneath the orbit (the bony cavity containing the eyeball)

subscapular below the scapula (shoulder blade)

substernal retractions indrawing beneath the sternum (breastbone)

supination turning the palm upward; moving the bones of the forearm so that the palm of the hand turns from posterior to anterior in the anatomic position

supine (supine position) lying on the back with the face upward; also called *dorsal position*

suppository a solid, cone-shaped, medicated substance inserted into the rectum, vagina, or urethra

supraclavicular retractions indrawing above the clavicles (collarbones)

suprapubic above the pubic arch

suprasternal retractions indrawing above the sternum

surfactant a lipoprotein mixture secreted in the alveoli that reduces surface tension of the fluid lining the alveoli

surgical asepsis measures that render and maintain objects free of all microorganisms including spores (sterile)

suture in surgery, a surgical stitch used to close accidental or surgical wounds; in anatomy, a junction line of the skull bones

symptoms (covert data) see *subjective data*

syncope fainting or temporary loss of consciousness

syndrome a group of signs and symptoms resulting from a single cause and constituting a typical clinical picture, such as the shock syndrome

synovial joint a freely movable joint surrounded by a capsule enclosing a cavity that contains a transparent, viscid fluid

syphilis a sexually transmitted disease caused by the microorganism *Treponema pallidum*

syringe an instrument used to inject or withdraw liquids

systemic pertaining to the body (or other system) as a whole

systole the period when the ventricles of the heart are contracted

systolic pressure the pressure of the blood against the arterial walls when the ventricles of the heart contract

tablet a medication in solid form that is compressed and molded

tachycardia an excessively rapid pulse or heart rate, over 100 beats per minute in an adult

tachypnea abnormally fast respirations, usually more than 24 per minute, marked by quick, shallow breaths

tactile (vocal) fremitus vibrations, palpable with the palms of the hands, originating in the larynx and transmitted to the chest wall during speech

T-binder a cloth in the shape of a T often used to retain dressings in the genital region

Td combined tetanus and diphtheria toxoid used for people over 6 years of age; it has less diphtheria toxoid than does DT

temporal pulse a pulse point where the temporal artery passes over the temporal bone of the skull

tenesmus straining; painful, ineffective straining during defecation or urination

tetany a syndrome manifested by muscle twitching, cramps, convulsions, and sharp flexion of the wrist and ankle joints

therapy treatment or remedy

thrombocytopenia an abnormal reduction in the number of platelets in the blood

thrombophlebitis inflammation of a vein followed by formation of a blood clot

thrombosis the development of a blood clot

thrombus a solid mass of blood constituents in the circulatory system; a clot (plural: thrombi)

tic a repetitive twitching of the muscles, often of the face or upper trunk

tidal volume the volume of air that is normally inhaled and exhaled

tinnitus a ringing or buzzing sensation in the ears

tissue perfusion supplying nutrients and oxygen to body tissues and organs

tomography a scanning procedure during which several x-ray beams pass through the body part from different angles

tonicity the normal condition of tension or tone, for example, of a muscle

tonus the slight, continual contraction of muscles

topical applied externally, for example, to the skin or mucous membranes

tortuous twisted

total lung capacity the maximum volume to which the lungs can be expanded

total parenteral nutrition administration of a hypertonic solution of carbohydrates, amino acids, and lipids by an indwelling intravenous catheter placed into the superior vena cava via the jugular or subclavian vein; also called *intravenous hyperalimentation*

tourniquet a device, such as a rubber strip, that is wrapped around a body area to compress the blood vessels

toxemia a generalized toxic state caused by the distribution of poisonous products of bacteria throughout the body

toxin a poison produced by some microorganisms, animals, and plants

tracheal tug an indrawing and downward pulling of the trachea during inhalation

tracheostomy procedure by which an opening is made in the anterior portion of the trachea and a cannula is introduced into the opening

traction the exertion of a pulling force

trademark (brand name) name of drug given by the drug manufacturer

transcutaneous electrical nerve stimulation (TENS) the placement of electrodes on the surface of the skin over a peripheral nerve pathway for the purpose of relieving pain

transfusion the introduction of whole blood or its components, such as serum, erythrocytes, or platelets, into the venous circulation

trapeze bar a triangular handgrip suspended from an overbed frame

trauma injury

tremor an involuntary muscle contraction, for example, quivering, twitching, or convulsions

Trendelenburg's position a bed position with the head of the bed lowered and the foot raised, while the bed foundation remains even; in some agencies, the position involves elevation of the knees, with the feet lowered and the head lowered

trocar a sharp, pointed instrument that fits inside a cannula and is used to pierce body cavities

trochanter either of two processes below the neck of the femur

trochanter roll a rolled towel support placed against the hips to prevent external rotation of the legs

troche a lozenge

tumor an uncontrolled and progressive growth of cells

tuning fork an instrument shaped like a two-pronged fork and made of metal; the prongs vibrate when struck

turgor normal cell tension; fullness

tympany a hollow, drumlike sound produced on percussion over organs that contain gas or air

ulcer a localized sloughing of skin tissue or mucous membrane commonly associated with varicosities or hyperactivity of the gastrointestinal tract

ultrasound high-frequency, mechanical, radiant energy

unconscious incapable of responding to sensory stimuli; insensible

unilateral affecting one side

unit dose system (of drugs) prepackaged and labeled individual doses of medication for each client; the amount of medication the client is to receive at a prescribed hour

universal donor a person with type O blood

universal recipient a person with type AB blood

unsterile containing microorganisms; unsterile material may be clean or contaminated

urea a substance found in urine, blood, and lymph; the main nitrogenous substance in blood

ureterostomy an artificial opening into the ureter

urethritis inflammation of the urethra

urgency (urinary) a feeling that one must urinate

urinal a receptacle used to collect urine

urinalysis a laboratory analysis of the urine

urinary diversion see *urostomy*

urobilinogen a colorless compound found in the intestines from the reduction of bilirubin

urostomy (ureterostomy, urinary diversion) an opening through the abdominal wall into the urinary tract that permits the drainage of urine

urticaria an allergic reaction marked by smooth, reddened, slightly elevated patches of skin and intense itching (hives)

uvula a small fleshy mass projecting from the soft palate above the base of the tongue

vaccine suspension of killed, attenuated, or living microorganisms administered to prevent or treat an infectious disease

Valsalva maneuver forceful exhalation against a closed glottis, which increases intrathoracic pressure

varicosity the state of having swollen, distended, and knotted veins, especially in the legs

vasectomy ligation and cutting of the vas deferens, rendering the male sterile

vasoconstriction a decrease in the caliber (lumen) of blood vessels

vasodilation an increase in the caliber (lumen) of blood vessels

vasopressor an agent that causes the blood pressure to rise

vasospasm spasm or constriction of the blood vessels

ventilation the movement of air; the act of breathing

ventral toward or at the front of; anterior

ventricle a small cavity, such as those located in the brain or the heart

vertigo dizziness

vesicular sounds normal, quiet, rustling, or swishing respiratory sounds heard over the terminal bronchioles and alveoli during auscultation

vial a glass medication container with a sealed rubber cap, for single or multiple doses

vibration a technique of rapidly agitating the hands while pressing on a body area

virulence the degree of strength or power of an organism to produce disease

virus minute infectious agent smaller than a bacterium

viscera large interior organs in body cavities, such as the liver and stomach (singular: viscus)

viscosity the quality of being viscous; the thickness or resistance of a fluid

vital capacity maximum amount of air that can be exhaled following a maximum inhalation

vital (cardinal) signs measurement of physiologic functioning—specifically, temperature, pulse, respirations, and blood pressure; may include pain and pulse oximetry

vitiligo patches of hypopigmented skin

vocal resonance vibrations of the larynx transmitted during speech through the respiratory system to the chest wall

void urinate, micturate

vomitus material vomited

walker a metal, rectangular frame used as an aid to ambulation

Weber's test a test that assesses bone conduction of sound

wheal see *bleb*

wheeze a whistling sound on exhalation that usually indicates narrowing of the bronchial air passages

xiphoid process the tip of the sternum

x-rays electromagnetic radiations with extremely short wavelengths (Roentgen rays)

INDEX

Page numbers followed by *f* indicate figures; numbers followed by *t* indicate tables; numbers followed by *b* indicate boxes.